Animal Biology and Care

Third Edition

Sue Dallas
VN, Certificate in Education

Emily Jewell MSc, BSc (Hons), Certificate in Education
Curriculum Area Manager in Animal Management
Reaseheath College
Nantwich
Cheshire

This edition first published 2014 © 2014 by John Wiley & Sons, Ltd

Registered Office

John Wiley & Sons, Ltd, The Atrium, Southern Gate, Chichester, West Sussex, PO19 8SQ, UK

Editorial Offices

9600 Garsington Road, Oxford, OX4 2DQ, UK

The Atrium, Southern Gate, Chichester, West Sussex, PO19 8SQ, UK

1606 Golden Aspen Drive, Suites 103 and 104, Ames, Iowa 50010, USA

For details of our global editorial offices, for customer services and for information about how to apply for permission to reuse the copyright material in this book please see our website at www.wiley.com/wiley-blackwell

The right of the author to be identified as the author of this work has been asserted in accordance with the UK Copyright, Designs and Patents Act 1988.

Library of Congress Cataloging-in-Publication Data

Dallas, S. E. (Sue E.), author.
   Animal biology and care / Sue Dallas, Emily Jewell. – Third edition.
      p. ; cm.
   Includes bibliographical references and index.
   ISBN 978-1-118-27606-8 (pbk.)
   I. Jewell, Emily, author.   II. Title.
   [DNLM: 1. Animal Diseases–nursing.   2. Animal Husbandry.   3. Animal Technicians.   4. Animals, Domestic–anatomy & histology.   5. Veterinary Medicine–methods. SF 774.5]
   SF745
   636.089–dc23

                              2014000060

A catalogue record for this book is available from the British Library.

Wiley also publishes its books in a variety of electronic formats. Some content that appears in print may not be available in electronic books.

Cover image: iStockphoto © AngiePhotos
Cover design by Steve Thompson

Set in 10/12pt Minion by SPi Publisher Services, Pondicherry, India
Printed and bound in Malaysia by Vivar Printing Sdn Bhd

1   2014

Animal Biology and Care

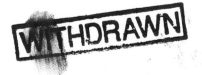

Contents

Preface

Having purchased this book when it was first published in 2000, it soon became an essential reference text for my students studying L2 and L3 programmes in Animal Care/Management as well as the intended market of those studying on Animal Nursing Assistant/Veterinary Care Assistant programmes. Now updated, I have aimed to ensure that the book remains a useful study companion to those undertaking such programmes now and in the future.

This book would also be useful for those working in the animal industry that need to enhance their knowledge in order to better manage the animals in their care.

The format of this latest edition aims to provide a logical flow through the chapters, following the same structural organisation of the previous editions. New photographs and additional diagrams have been included to enhance learning. Each chapter now has a learning outcome summary for readers to check their knowledge and understanding at the end of each chapter. To support the content of the book, online questions have also been developed to check and support learning.

Emily Jewell
MSc, BSc (Hons), Certificate in Education
Curriculum Area Manager in Animal Management
Reaseheath College
Nantwich
Cheshire

Acknowledgments

I am grateful to the staff at Wiley for their help during the writing of this edition, particularly Jessica Evans whose guidance and patience has been unending and much appreciated. My thanks also go to the tutor (Lisa Gee RVN) and students of the L3 Diploma in Veterinary Nursing at Reaseheath College for agreeing to coax the animals into the relevant positions for the new photographs. As always, thanks go to my family for their continuing support and encouragement. Finally, to you the reader, I hope that this new edition remains as well used as previous ones.

Emily Jewell
MSc, BSc (Hons), Certificate in Education
Curriculum Area Manager in Animal Management
Reaseheath College
Nantwich
Cheshire

Companion Website

This book is accompanied by a companion website:

www.wiley.com/go/dallas/animal-biology-care

The website includes:

- Almost 200 interactive Multiple Choice Questions organized by chapter so that you can test your knowledge
- Chapter summaries providing learning objectives for each chapter
- PowerPoints of all figures from the book for downloading (a password is required, which can be found in the book)

Section 1
Animal Biology

Chapter 1
Cells and Basic Tissues

Summary

In this chapter, the learning outcomes are:

- To understand the essential functions required to sustain life – MRS GREN
- To be able to identify the structure and function of animal cells and tissues
- To be able to recognize the diversity of animal cells and tissues in existence

What is Biology?

Biology is the study of life and living organisms

What is life?

In order to be considered as a living organism, an organism must be able to perform all the following essential functions of life:

- *Movement* – the organism is capable of moving itself or a part of itself.
- *Reproduction* – the organism is capable of reproducing itself so that the species doesn't die out.
- *Sensitivity* – to stimuli in its surroundings in order to avoid life-threatening occurrences in the environment.
- *Growth* – sustained growth from within by a process which involves the intake of new materials from the outside and their incorporation into the internal structure of the organism.
- *Release of energy from respiration* – in a controlled manner and in a form usable by the organism. The process of respiration releases energy from food to sustain life.
- *Excretion* – the removal of the waste products of metabolism from the organism.
- *Nutrition* – taking in food materials which provide energy to maintain life and growth.

Animal Biology and Care, Third Edition. Sue Dallas and Emily Jewell.
© 2014 John Wiley & Sons, Ltd. Published 2014 by John Wiley & Sons, Ltd.
Companion Website: www.wiley.com/go/dallas/animal-biology-care

The cell is the simplest functional unit of all tissues and has the ability to perform individually all the essential life functions. Organisms may be single-celled or multi-celled. Within the multicellular organisms, the constituent cells show a wide range of specialisations. Cells can be viewed as the building blocks of the body, and so the following can be said:

- *Cells* form…
- *Tissues*, and tissues form…
- *Organs*, and organs… join together to form *systems* within the body.
- Systems have a specific function to perform in the living organism.

The diversity of cells

Cells are not all identical (Fig. 1.1) but all have the same basic structure. Each component of a cell is known as an organelle:

- *Cell membrane* – the surrounding membrane of the cell which encloses the cytoplasm and is only 0.00001 mm in thickness. The cell membrane is the outer boundary that controls all exchanges between the cell and its surrounding environment. The cell membrane allows certain chemicals to pass in and out of the cell either by *diffusion, osmosis* or *active transport*. The cell membrane is described as being *selectively permeable*.

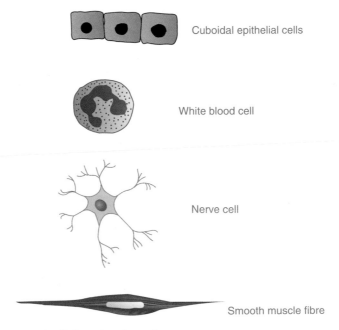

Fig. 1.1 Diversity of cells from their basic form.

- *Nucleus* – acts as the cell's brain and controls the cell's activities and there is usually only one nucleus in the cell. The nucleus also contains the chromosomes.
- *Cytoplasm* – a jelly-like material that supports the organelles within the cell. It contains enzymes and many other chemicals that aid cell metabolism.
- *Chromosomes* – rod-shaped components that contain the hereditary information of the organism. Chromosomes contain deoxyribonucleic acid (DNA) which controls the characteristics that an organism inherits from its parents.
- *Mitochondria* – the energy-producing organelles where cell respiration takes place.
- *Endoplasmic reticulum* (ER) – is a series of tubules acting as a transport and packaging system. ER may be rough ER or smooth ER. Rough ER has ribosomes attached to it where proteins are synthesized. This protein can be used by the cell to synthesize enzymes and hormones. Smooth ER has no ribosomes and is used to synthesize and transport lipids (fats) and steroids made within the body.
- *Ribosomes* – build proteins within the cell which are then joined to form amino acids which are essential to growth. Ribosomes contain *ribonucleic acid* (RNA).
- *Centrosome* – an area found near the nucleus and made up of two *centrioles*. Centrioles are important during cell division and the formation of the cilia and flagella of certain cells (the slender projecting hairs for movement of single-celled organisms). Centrioles can only be seen during cell division; otherwise, a dark area known as the centrosome is observed.
- *Lysosomes* – are dark round bodies containing enzymes responsible for splitting complex chemical compounds into simpler ones (known as *lysis*, meaning 'to break up') followed by digestion. They also destroy worn-out organelles within the cell. These destructive enzymes are packaged in an area of the cell called the *Golgi complex* or *Golgi body*.
- *Peroxisomes* – are similar to lysosomes but they contain a different type of enzyme that breaks down toxic materials in the cell. Peroxisomes are good at breaking down fatty acids, alcohol and hydrogen peroxide made during digestion.

The organelles listed earlier are common to virtually all cells, but the shape, form and contents of individual cells show much variation. The structural characteristics of a particular cell are closely related to its functions (Fig. 1.2).

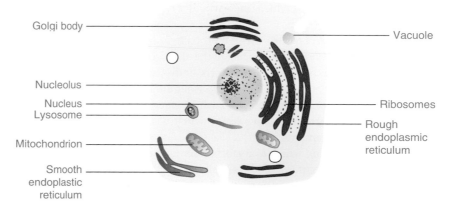

Fig. 1.2   Basic cell structure.

Types of cell found in the animal body

- *Epithelial cells* – have a shape and form that make them most suitable for lining the surface of the body and the organs and cavities within it.
- *Glandular cells* – are responsible for producing some kind of secretion, for example, mucus, to lubricate between tissues.
- *Osteoblasts* – produce bone tissue.
- *Erythrocytes* (*red blood cells*) – have a shape designed to hold the red pigment haemoglobin which conveys oxygen around the body. In order to do this, they are one of the few cells in the body which no longer contain a nucleus.
- *Nerve cells* – or neurones have slender armlike processes which will transmit electrical impulses through the nervous system to reach the whole body.
- *Muscle cells* – are also capable of electrical activity accompanied by a muscle contraction for body movement.
- *Sperm cells* – are the male sex cells. They have a tail for swimming and only contain half the amount of chromosomes.
- *Ova* – are the female sex cells. They contain only half the amount of chromosomes of other cells in the body.

Cells

No matter what the type of cell found in an organism, cells have needs that must be met in order to survive:

- Food for energy
- Water (body fluid) to hydrate the cells
- Oxygen to all cells
- A suitable temperature in which to live

Animal Tissues

Tissues are a collection of cells and their products which have a common fundamental function and in which one particular type of cell predominates:

- *Epithelial tissue* – forms a protective layer both inside and on the surface of the body. Examples of this tissue are the skin, glands and linings of the various body systems.
- *Connective tissue* – supports body tissues and acts as a transport system to move materials vital to tissue cells around the body. Examples of this tissue are:
  - *loose connective tissue* which surrounds organs
  - *dense connective tissue* which has great strength and is found as tendons and ligaments
  - *blood* which transports essential nutrients, gases, waste products, hormones and enzymes to and from all body cells
  - *cartilage* and *bone* which provide shape and protection for organs and allow movement.

- *Muscular tissue* – are concerned with movement of the skeleton, the organ systems and the heart.
- *Nervous tissue* – is concerned with transporting messages to tissues and connecting the body as a whole for the required response.

Epithelial tissue

This tissue covers all surfaces of the body, both inside and out, whether it is a surface, a cavity or a tube. It is made up of a diverse group of tissues which are involved in a wide range of activities such as secretion of a special fluid, protection and absorption.

Depending on their function, the cells of this tissue will have varied shape, structure and thickness. Epithelial tissues are classified according to appearance:

- *Number of layers* – a single layer of these cells is called *simple epithelium*; more than one layer is called *stratified epithelium*.
- *Shape* of the cells involved.
- *Specialisations*, such as tiny hairs called cilia or special thickened surface tissue called keratin, which covers the nose and pads of the feet.
- *Glandular* – means that it is involved in secretion. Secretions which go directly into the bloodstream are called *hormones* and are produced by glands of the *endocrine* or *ductless system*. Some secretions are produced by glands that have ducts. The secretion is released through the duct onto the surface of the cell. Glands with ducts belong to the exocrine system and an example of this is when enzymes are produced by the pancreas.

Types of epithelial tissue

Epithelial tissue has many different functions, and this therefore reflects in the different forms that can be found. There are six main types of epithelial tissue:

- *Pavement* – can be found lining the surfaces involved in the transport of gases (lungs) or fluids (walls of blood vessels) (Fig. 1.3a).
- *Cuboidal* – can be found lining small ducts and tubes such as those of the kidney, pancreas and salivary glands of the mouth (Fig. 1.3b).
- *Columnar* – located on highly absorbing surfaces like the small intestine for the uptake of nutrients (Fig. 1.3c).
- *Ciliated* – has tiny hair-like projections in parallel rows on the surface of the cell, which beat in a wave-like manner, moving films of mucus or fluid in a particular direction. For example, in the respiratory airway (trachea), they remove unwanted inhaled materials (Fig. 1.4a).
- *Glandular* – which secrete a special fluid containing hormones or enzymes (Fig. 1.4b).
- *Stratified* – this type of epithelium has two or more layers of cells. Its function is mostly protection. It can be found lining the mouth or as skin (Fig. 1.4c).

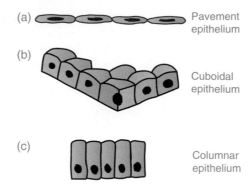

Fig. 1.3 Pavement, cuboidal and columnar tissue.

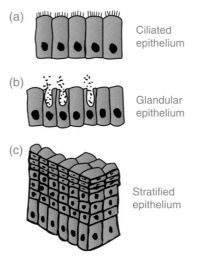

Fig. 1.4 Ciliated, glandular and stratified tissues.

Connective tissue

Connective tissue binds all the other body tissues together. It supports them and acts as a transport system for the exchange of nutrients, metabolites and waste products between tissues and the circulatory system (Fig. 1.5).

Connective tissues occur in many different forms with a wide range of physical properties:

- *Loose connective tissue* acts as a type of packing material between other tissues with specific functions.
- *Dense connective tissue* provides tough support in the skin.
- *Rigid* forms of connective tissue, like cartilage and bone, support the skeleton.

Connective tissue also has functions including the storage of fat in adipose tissue, fighting infection and tissue repair.

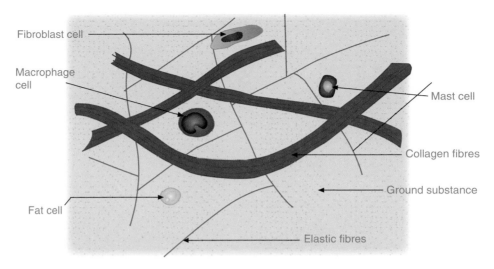

Fig. 1.5 Connective tissue.

Connective tissue has two components:

(1) *Cells*:
    (a) fibroblasts for repair and maintenance of the tissue
    (b) fat-storing cells
    (c) defence and immune function cells called *macrophages*.
(2) *Ground substance* – a material which holds together other materials to make up tissue and looks like a semi-fluid gel.

Connective tissue can be described as a mixture of fibres in different proportions. Its efficiency in binding structures together is achieved by the special grouping of proteins in the ground substance. The particular type and abundance of fibre present depend on the stresses and strains to which the tissue is normally subjected.

Connective tissue is composed of two types of fibre:

• *Collagen* – produced by the fibroblasts and is not elastic but has great tensile strength. Tendons by which muscles are attached to the bones are composed of collagen fibres.
• *Elastin* – has great elasticity and is found in ligaments which bind the bones of the skeleton together.

Blood

Blood is a highly specialised tissue consisting of several types of cell suspended in a fluid medium called *plasma* (Fig. 1.6). The cellular constituents consist of:

• Red blood cells (erythrocytes)
• White blood cells (leucocytes)
• Platelets (thrombocytes)

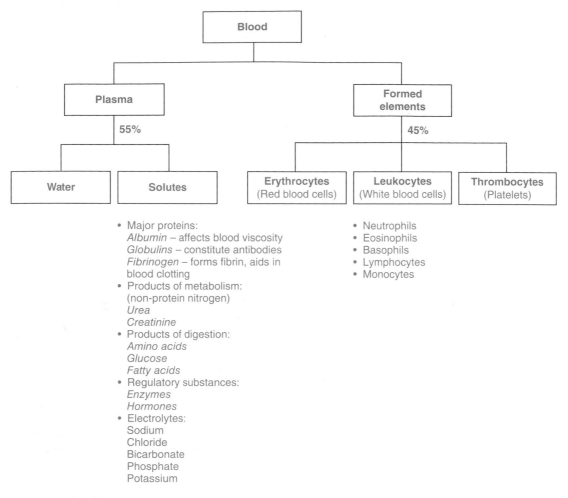

Fig. 1.6 Blood components.

Blood has a varied structure and performs a wide range of functions. One of its main functions is the transportation of red blood cells and all materials in the plasma around the body. Blood is considered a tissue because it connects all the cells in the body together.

Living animals constantly absorb useful substances like oxygen and food, which must then be distributed throughout their bodies. They produce a continuous stream of waste materials, such as carbon dioxide, which must be removed from their bodies before they reach harmful levels. The distribution of food, oxygen and other substances throughout the body and the removal of any wastes are performed by this transport system tissue.

Composition of the blood

Fluid called *plasma* makes up about 60%. Cells and other material in transit make up the remaining 40%.

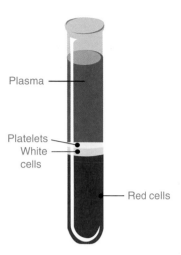

Plasma

Platelets
White
cells

Red cells

Fig. 1.7   Blood separated into layers.

If a sample of blood (mixed with an anticoagulant to stop it from clotting) was put into a centrifuge and spun to separate out the component parts, it would show at the top of the tube the fluid part (plasma), then the platelets (cell fragments), then the white blood cells and finally the red cells (Fig. 1.7).

Plasma – is mainly water containing a variety of dissolved substances which are transported from one part of the body to another. To give a few examples, food materials (glucose, lipids and amino acids) are conveyed from the small intestine to the liver, urea from the liver to the kidneys and hormones from various ductless glands to their target organs. Cells are constantly shedding materials into the blood which flows past them and removing materials from it. Plasma provides the medium through which this continual exchange takes place.

PLASMA	SERUM
Fibrinogen (protein for clotting) **plus** water, protein, glucose, lipids, amino acids, salts, enzymes, hormones and waste products	Contains water, protein, glucose, lipids, amino acids, salts, enzymes, hormones and waste products **but** no proteins for clotting (these have been used up)

Plasma carries many more products than the diagram shows, including the plasma proteins called albumin, globulin and fibrinogen. Fibrinogen plays an important role in the process of blood clotting. When it has been used up by clot formation, then the fluid part of blood seen at the site of injury is called *serum*. Therefore, the serum is plasma with the fibrinogen removed. About 92% of blood is made of water, and this same water can be forced into the tissues. It is then called *tissue fluid* because of its location.

It is important to realise that plasma and the tissue fluid derived from it form the environment which keeps body cells alive. In a sense, these fluids are equivalent to a pond or fish

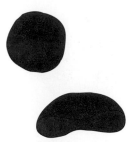

Fig. 1.8   Cross section of a red blood cell showing its biconcave shape.

tank in which both single-celled organisms and multi-celled organisms live and are supplied with their food and oxygen and into which they excrete waste.

Red blood cells (erythrocytes)

These are produced in the red or active bone marrow. The main function of red blood cells is to carry oxygen from the respiratory organ to the tissues, and their structure is modified accordingly. These cells have had their nucleus removed, with the result that the cell is sunk in on each side, giving it the shape of a biconcave disc. It is surrounded by a thin elastic membrane, and the interior of the cell is filled with the red pigment haemoglobin which combines with and carries oxygen (Fig. 1.8).

White blood cells (leucocytes)

The white cells are fewer in number and have a very different role to play. They fall into two groups (Fig. 1.9):

- *Granulocytes (granules in the cytoplasm)*. These are produced in the bone marrow.
    - *Neutrophils* – phagocytic cells
    - *Eosinophils* – respond to allergies
    - *Basophils* – promote inflammation for healing of tissue
- *Agranulocytes (no granules in their cytoplasm)*. Produced in the bone marrow or lymph system.
    - *Lymphocytes* – support the immune system
    - *Monocytes* – phagocyte cells

Phagocyte or phagocytic means 'cell eater'. These cells eat or engulf other cells/materials that may be harmful and destroy them. Red cells will remain in the bloodstream to perform their role of oxygen carrier, but white cells will only use the bloodstream as a transporter from their site of origin to the capillaries where they will push through the wall of the blood vessel and into the tissue spaces. Those that are phagocytic will gather in and around wounds and destroy bacteria and any other harmful materials. In this manner, the cells assist in 'fighting infection'.

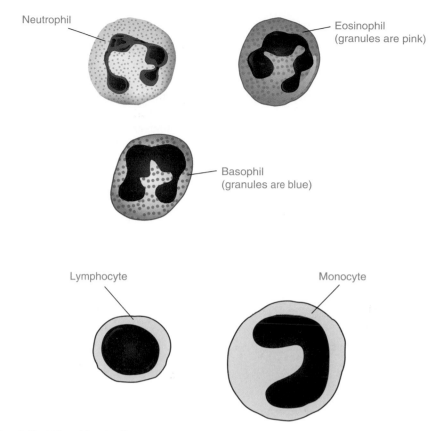

Fig. 1.9 White blood cells.

Bone and cartilage

There are two kinds of skeletal tissue, bone and cartilage.

Bone

Bone tissue is closely related to connective tissue in that it consists of cells embedded in an organic matrix (ground substance). However, this matrix is comparatively hard. The cells of the bone are called *osteoblasts* and *osteoclasts*.

Cartilage

Cartilage is a dense, clear, blue/white material which provides support for the body and can be elastic or rigid. Found mainly in the joints, it has no blood vessels but is covered by a membrane called the *perichondrium* from which it receives its blood supply. The cells of cartilage are called *chondroblasts*.

There are three types of cartilage:

(1) *Hyaline cartilage* – the cells for hyaline production are called *chondro-cytes*. They lie within a hyaline matrix with collagen fibres running through. Hyaline is a smooth tissue and forms articular joint surfaces for the bones and the C-shaped rings of cartilage that keep the trachea open for air passage into the lungs.

(2) *Fibrocartilage* – this is stronger than hyaline but with a similar base structure that contains more collagen fibres. It surrounds the articular surface of some bones, for example, in the hip joint (acetabulum) and the shoulder joint (gle-noid cavity), and is also found in the stifle or knee joint as pads of cartilage called *menisci*.

(3) *Elastic* – this has a hyaline matrix and many elastic fibres which provide its elastic properties. It is found in the ear flap (pinna) and in the larynx area of the throat.

Muscular tissue

Muscular tissue has a well-developed ability to contract due to its structure. Muscle cells are usually long, thin and thread-like and are often called *fibres*. There are three main types of fibres:

- *Skeletal* (also called voluntary and striated) (Fig. 1.10)
- *Smooth* (also called involuntary, nonstriated and visceral) (Fig. 1.11)
- *Cardiac* (Fig. 1.12)

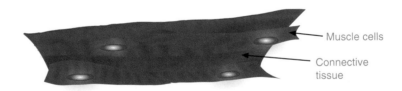

Fig. 1.10 Skeletal (striated) muscle fibre.

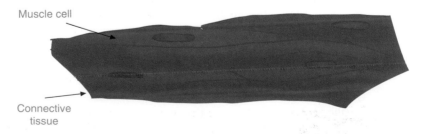

Fig. 1.11 Smooth (non-striated) muscle fibre.

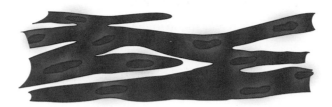

Fig. 1.12 Cardiac muscle fibre.

Skeletal muscle

Skeletal muscle is located in muscles attached to the skeleton. The cells are cylindrical and vary from about 1 mm to 5 cm in length. Since skeletal muscles respond to the will of the animal, the cells are also called *voluntary* muscle cells.

Skeletal muscles are formed of parallel muscle cells (*fibres*) held together in small bundles by connective tissue. These are collected into larger groups, enclosed in connective tissue which ultimately form the muscle and are surrounded by yet more connective tissue commonly called the *muscle sheath*.

When muscles are close to one another, the sheaths may thicken to form *intermuscular septa*.

All the connective tissue within and around the muscles continues into the connective tissue of the structure to which the muscle is attached, i.e. bone. Sometimes, the muscle appears to attach directly, but usually, the connective tissue leaves the muscle as a fibrous band known as a *tendon* (i.e. Achilles tendon on the point of the hock) or as a fibrous sheet called an *aponeurosis* (i.e. the sheet of muscle and connective tissue called the diaphragm).

Some muscles are named according to their shape, some according to their functions and others according to their position in the body.

Under the microscope, skeletal muscle cells look striped (they have *striations*), and so, this type of muscle tissue may also be referred to as striated muscle.

Smooth muscle

Smooth muscle is specialized for continuous contractions of little force but over a greater section of muscle tissue. This is in direct contrast to skeletal muscle, which is specialized for relatively forceful contractions of short duration and under voluntary control. Smooth muscle, for example, is found in the intestinal wall and contracts in continuous rhythm, moving food through the tract by *peristaltic action*.

Smooth muscle fibres are spindle shaped and about 0.5 mm in length or shorter. Under the microscope, they look smooth. Only small amounts of connective tissue bind them together to form sheets or layers of muscle tissue. They may also be called *involuntary* muscles because they are not controlled by the will of the animal. These fibres are found in the muscle of organs, hence the alternative name of *visceral* muscle.

Cardiac muscle

Cardiac muscle is only found in the heart. It produces strong contractions using a lot of energy but its contractions are continuous. In order for continuous contraction to take place, the fibres have junctions or connections with the surrounding fibres which allow very rapid contractions of all nearby tissue. The cells are elongated and are the only muscle cells which frequently branch. They are held together by very small amounts of connective tissue.

Nervous tissue

The function of nervous tissue is to transmit electrical messages from one part of the body to another. As a result of this, nerve cells are interconnected in a very complex way. The cells can transmit and sometimes store information because of this complex link-up with each other.

Nerve cells are called *neurones* (Fig. 1.13), and they connect and communicate to form pathways so that the body can respond to information received. Neurones vary in size and shape depending on where they are in the nervous system. However, all neurones have the same basic structure. They consist of a large cell body containing the nucleus surrounded by cytoplasm, with two types of processes extending from the cell body: a single axon and one or more dendrites:

- *Dendrites* are branched, tapering processes which either end in specialized *sense receptors* (information) or form junctions (*synapses*) with neighbouring neurones from which they receive electrical stimuli, which are passed to the cells beyond.
- *Axons* extend from the cell body as a tube-like structure of variable length, carrying stimuli or messages away to the next nerve cell.

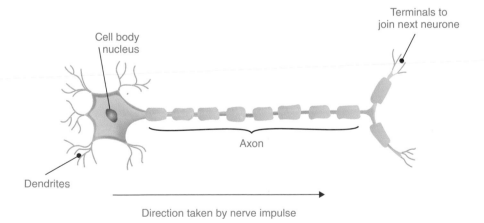

Fig. 1.13 A neurone.

Chapter 2
Movement of Materials within the Body

Summary

In this chapter, the learning outcomes are:

- To identify and be able to describe the following transport processes in the body:
  - Diffusion
  - Osmosis
  - Phagocytosis
  - Active transport
- To identify the structure and function of the lymphatic system

In Chapter 1, it was stated that substances can move in and out of cells through the semipermeable membrane of the cell. This chapter will focus on how this happens.

The exchange of substances in and out of the cell can occur via one of the following processes:

(1) Diffusion
(2) Osmosis
(3) Phagocytosis
(4) Active transport

Diffusion

Diffusion is the process of movement of molecules from a region where they are at a comparatively high concentration to a region where they are at a lower concentration. No energy is needed for the process of diffusion to successfully take place. Diffusion continues until the molecules are uniformly distributed throughout the system. This process is very important in the movement of molecules and salts (electrolytes or ions) in and out of cells. An example of where diffusion occurs in the animal body is gas exchange in the cell. All cells need oxygen to live. Oxygen is continually being used up in cell respiration

Animal Biology and Care, Third Edition. Sue Dallas and Emily Jewell.
© 2014 John Wiley & Sons, Ltd. Published 2014 by John Wiley & Sons, Ltd.
Companion Website: www.wiley.com/go/dallas/animal-biology-care

which takes place in the mitochondria, and so, the concentration of oxygen inside the cell will be lower than it is in the blood and tissue fluids as a result. Oxygen molecules will diffuse into the cell from outside. With carbon dioxide, the reverse is true: its concentration is highest inside the cells, where it is continually being formed. This results in carbon dioxide molecules diffusing out of the cells.

Anything that increases the concentration of a substance in the body will favour diffusion. Blood is involved here to carry away the diffused substance, so encouraging further diffusion.

Osmosis

Osmosis is the movement of water through a semipermeable membrane while expending no energy (Fig. 2.1).

Although the cell wall membrane is fully permeable to respiratory gases, it is not permeable to all substances. The nature of the membrane means that only molecules that are small enough will diffuse through it unimpeded. Larger molecules either penetrate slowly or not at all. The membrane is therefore called semipermeable, permitting the passage of some substances but not others.

Osmosis is really a special case of diffusion: it involves the passage of water molecules from a region of high concentration to a region of lower concentration. The concentration will be supplied by other products like salts.

Large molecules cannot pass through the membrane, but water passes through easily.

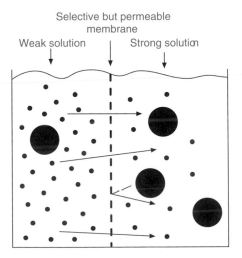

Fig. 2.1 Osmosis.

Terms relating to osmosis

- *Osmosis* – is the diffusion of fluid through a selectively permeable membrane, from where water is in a high concentration (a weak solution) to where water is in a low concentration (a strong solution). *Osmotic pressure* helps to keep fluid in its correct compartment within the body.
- *Isotonic* – refers to solutions which cause no transfer of fluid either into or out of a cell. These are the solutions most frequently used in fluid replacement in sick animals, such as 0.9% sodium chloride.
- *Hypertonic* – these are solutions with an osmotic pressure higher than that of body fluids. If the cell is surrounded by a solution with an osmotic pressure higher than that of the cell, water passes out of the cell, causing it to shrink.
- *Hypotonic* – these are solutions with an osmotic pressure lower than body fluid. In this case, the cell is surrounded by almost pure water which allows water to enter cells by osmosis, causing the cell to swell and even to burst.

Phagocytosis

Large molecules are unable to cross the cell membrane via diffusion or osmosis. This is achieved by specialized cells which are able to 'cell eat' or *phagocytose*. This process was mentioned when discussing white blood cells which take up and destroy bacteria and other particles which could be harmful to the body.

To phagocytose, the cell membrane changes shape to form a flask-like depression enclosing the particles. The neck of the depression then closes and seals itself off as a food vacuole and migrates towards the centre of the cell. The material is digested by enzymes within the cell. Any useful food products resulting from this process are absorbed into the cell cytoplasm. Phagocytosis is a selective process with the cell distinguishing between food particles and harmful materials.

Active transport

Diffusion is a purely physical process in which molecules or salts move from a region of higher to a region of lower concentration. But there are certain biological situations where the reverse happens: molecules or salts move from a region of low concentration to a region of higher concentration; i.e. they move against the concentration gradient. This process is known as *active transport*, and it will only take place in a living system that is actively producing energy by respiration. Active transport requires the cell to use energy as it is a very active process rather than a passive one.

Body fluid

Body fluid is not just made up of water. It is a fluid containing dissolved essential salts called electrolytes or ions. They are called electrolytes because they carry one or more electrical charges. Those that are positively charged are called cations, i.e. sodium and potassium. Those that are negatively charged are called anions, i.e. chloride and bicarbonate.

The role of electrolytes is to:

- Help control the osmotic pressure
- Assist the pH and buffer mechanisms
- Support the enzyme systems

About 60% of the body consists of fluids, and body fluid can be divided into two main areas:

- Intracellular fluid – 40%
- Extracellular fluid – 20%

Extracellular fluid is further divided into:

- Tissue fluid (interstitial) which bathes the tissues and cells
- Plasma, which is the water part of blood, needed to transport the cells, nutrients, gases, hormones and waste products

Acids and bases in the body

The acidity of a solution is expressed as its pH (per hydrogen). A pH of 7.0 represents neutral. A solution with a pH of less than 7.0 is acidic, and the lower the figure, the higher the acidity (the greater the hydrogen ion concentration). A solution whose pH is greater than 7.0 is basic or alkaline, and the higher the figure, the more basic is the solution.

The cells of the body function within a normal range of 7.35–7.45 pH. This normal range must be maintained by the body systems at all times for the correct internal environment.

Tissue fluid and the lymphatic system

Each tissue and organ in the body contains a dense network of capillaries (blood vessels that are one cell thick). These are called the capillary beds. Tissue fluid is forced under pressure through the capillary walls. This process tends to occur at the artery end of the capillary bed, since blood pressure is greatest at this point.

When tissue fluid is being forced out of the capillaries, the capillary wall acts as a filter holding back the red blood cells, most of the white cells and large protein molecules.

Substances which do pass through the capillary wall include:

- Water
- Oxygen
- Glucose
- Fatty acids

- Amino acids
- Vitamins and minerals
- Hormones and enzymes

Tissue fluid flows away from the capillaries and passes among the body cells, which extract oxygen, nutrients and other requirements from it and at the same time release carbon dioxide and other waste materials into it.

The lymphatic system

The lymphatic system consists of a system of open-ended tubes within the capillary bed areas, as numerous as the blood capillaries. The lymphatic system transports a fluid around the body. This fluid is called lymph.

Lymph is tissue fluid which is not absorbed back into the bloodstream after carrying required substances to the cells. This tissue fluid drains into the open-ended tubes of the lymph system known as lymph vessels. The structure of these vessels is similar to that of veins, in that they have a valve system to make sure fluid only flows in one direction. The movement of lymph in these vessels is achieved by the movement of surrounding tissues which squeeze or 'milk' the fluid in the lymph vessels.

At intervals in the lymphatic system, there are lymph nodes (Fig. 2.2), some of which are located near to the surface of the skin (Fig. 2.3). These structures contain a

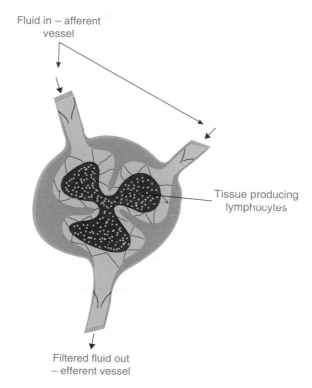

Fluid in – afferent vessel

Tissue producing lymphocytes

Filtered fluid out – efferent vessel

Fig. 2.2 Lymph node.

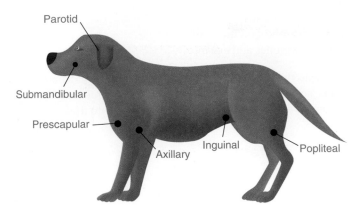

Fig. 2.3   Surface nodes.

system of narrow channels through which the lymph fluid will drain and be filtered. This filtering is assisted by phagocytic white blood cells, therefore filtering harmful substances out of the lymph, making the fluid safe enough to return to the main blood circulation.

Where this fluid returns into the bloodstream, lymph ducts can be found. From the right side of the head, neck and right forelimb, lymph drains via the right lymphatic duct. From the rest of the body, lymph drains via a collecting area called the *cisterna chyli* into the thoracic duct in the thorax or chest. This fluid will contain:

- Fats from the digestive system
- Water
- Electrolytes
- White blood cells
- Antibodies

Functions of the lymphatic system

The lymphatic system has several functions in the body:

- Return excess tissue fluid to the blood.
- Add lymphocytes (white blood cells) to the blood for the immune protection of the body.
- Absorb fats in the lacteals of the villi in the small intestine and carry them to the bloodstream.
- Filter out bacteria and other harmful substances via the nodes.

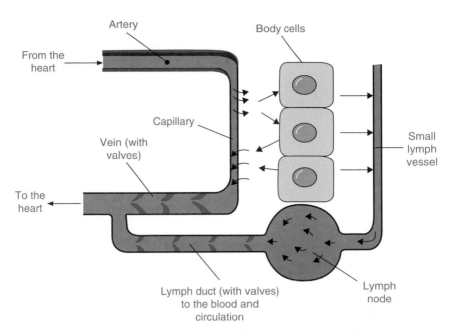

Fig. 2.4 Fluid movement from blood to lymph and back to blood.

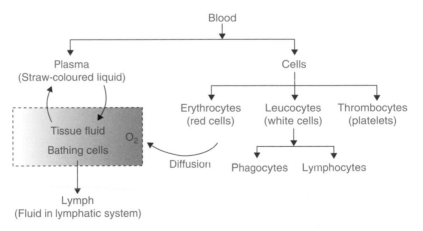

Fig. 2.5 Constituents of blood and their functions.

The lymphatic system is complementary to the blood and circulation system. Between them, they move fluid and other substances through the tissue spaces and help to keep the internal environment of the body within normal limits for healthy functioning (Figs. 2.4 and 2.5).

Chapter 3
Body Systems and Functions

Summary

In this chapter, the learning outcomes are:

- To identify the structure, function and interrelationships between body systems including:
  - ○ Circulatory system
  - ○ Respiratory system
  - ○ Digestive system
  - ○ Urinary system
  - ○ Nervous system
  - ○ Central nervous system
  - ○ Peripheral nervous system
  - ○ Endocrine system
  - ○ Sensory organs
  - ○ Integumentary system
  - ○ Skeletal system
  - ○ Reproductive system
- To define the term homeostasis and explain its importance in the body

The circulatory system

The circulatory system is a major system of the animal body. It is made up of:

- A pump – the **heart**
- A circuit of tubes which leave the pump, permeate the body and return to the pump – these tubes are the **arteries, veins and capillaries**

For the cells of a body to survive, they need for a supply of oxygen and nutrients that is replenished rapidly. Waste substances also need to be removed quickly to avoid

Animal Biology and Care, Third Edition. Sue Dallas and Emily Jewell.
© 2014 John Wiley & Sons, Ltd. Published 2014 by John Wiley & Sons, Ltd.
Companion Website: www.wiley.com/go/dallas/animal-biology-care

them building up in the body. In order for both of these processes to be achieved, the body needs an active supply and removal system. This is provided by the pump, the heart, which is connected to other systems in the body and therefore capable of responding as required to the needs of the tissues.

The circulatory system connects to all tissues and body cells and will transport:

- *Nutrients* – sugars, fats, amino acids, vitamins, minerals and salts
- *Oxygen*
- *Hormones* – chemical messages controlling the metabolism and development of the body and its operation as a unit
- *White blood cells* – which provide a defence system for the protection of the body

It will also:

- *Provide a clotting mechanism* – to prevent loss of blood from minor damage to the blood vessels
- *Carry heat* – to and from the cells and tissues depending on their requirements
- *Remove waste products* – such as carbon dioxide and other nitrogenous waste like urea and creatinine
- *Carry water* – to replenish the tissues and transport materials in the circulation

Blood vessels

There are several types of blood vessels in the body. Along with arteries, veins and capillaries are arterioles and venules. This section will focus on the first three.

Arteries

- Carry blood away from the heart.
- Carry oxygenated blood (except for the pulmonary artery to the lungs).
- Have thick muscular walls to assist with the movement of blood.
- Under high pressure, from heart muscle contractions.

Veins

- Carry blood towards the heart.
- Carry deoxygenated blood (except the pulmonary vein from the lungs to the heart).
- Have thin walls.
- Blood moved under low pressure and by the action of surrounding tissues.
- Have a valve system to prevent backflow of the blood (Fig. 3.1)

Capillaries

- Carry blood from arteries to veins.
- Blood movement is very slow to allow maximum diffusion of substances.

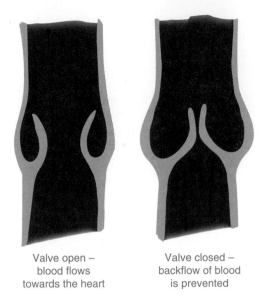

Valve open –
blood flows
towards the heart

Valve closed –
backflow of blood
is prevented

Fig. 3.1   Valve system in the veins to prevent backflow of the blood.

- Only one cell thick.
- Connects all cells and tissues, called capillary beds.
- Narrow, may only be wide enough for one blood cell at a time to pass through.

Location names for blood vessels

The larger blood vessels in the body have a name. For example, the main artery leaving the left side of the heart is called the *aorta*. Whenever the aorta divides to supply an organ, it takes a location name in order to assist anatomists to describe where they are in the body. An example of this would be the aortic division to supply the kidney with blood, called the *renal artery*. When blood leaves the kidney, the vessel is called the *renal vein*, and this will rejoin the main vein, the *vena cava*.

Consider where the following blood vessels may be located in the body:

- Cardiac artery
- Pulmonary artery
- Carotid artery
- Coronary
- Hepatic vein
- Femoral vein
- Cephalic vein
- Tibial vein

The heart

The heart (Fig. 3.2) lies between the two sides of the chest (the thorax), surrounded by the lungs, and is held in place by a structure called the *mediastinum*. It is made up of

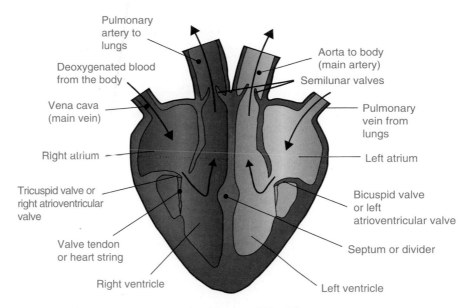

Fig. 3.2 The heart. Arrows indicate the direction of blood flow.

cardiac muscle which is a specialised type of muscle. Cardiac muscle differs from other types of muscles in three ways:

(1) It is comprised of branching muscle fibres connected to each other in the form of a network. This enables contractions to begin at one point in the heart and spread outwards in all directions.

(2) Heart or cardiac muscle contracts and relaxes rhythmically in 'beats'. The rhythm is generated within the muscle itself and not by impulses from the nervous system.

(3) Heart muscle does not get tired, despite continuous and rapid contractions over many years.

The mammalian heart consists of two pumps fused together, each of which has two chambers:

- Right atrium and right ventricle
- Left atrium and left ventricle

The right side of the heart is the less muscular side, and it is responsible for pumping deoxygenated blood received from the body to the lungs for reoxygenation. The left side of the heart is very muscular and is responsible for pumping oxygenated blood received from the lungs to the body (Fig. 3.3). The blood pumped from the left side of the heart is under considerably high pressure, and this will ensure:

- Fast supply of materials to the cells and tissues
- Pushing of fluid from the circulation into the tissues

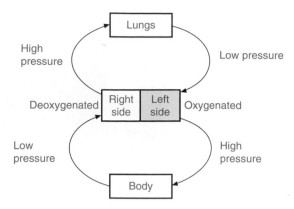

Fig. 3.3 The heart pump.

The heart is surrounded by a thick fibrous bag called the *pericardium*. Blood enters the heart from the body (systemic circulation) via the great veins, the *vena cava*, caudal and cranial vessels. The right atrium contracts to top up the right ventricle. When the right ventricle pumps, it pushes blood out through the pulmonary artery into the lungs (deoxygenated blood). After oxygenation of the blood in the lungs, the blood returns via the pulmonary veins to the left atrium. The left atrium then contracts to pump the blood through to the left ventricle. The left ventricle is the most muscular chamber of the heart, in order to be able to pump blood around the rest of the body via the *aorta*.

To stop blood flowing backwards (in the wrong direction), there are valves within the heart. On the *right* side of the heart, there are the:

- Right atrioventricular valve, also called the tricuspid valve
- Semilunar valve, also called the pulmonary semilunar valve

and on the *left* side of the heart, there are the:

- Left atrioventricular valve, also called the bicuspid or mitral valve
- Semilunar valve, also called aortic semilunar valve

At the base of the aorta, just above the semilunar valves, are the entrances to the left and right coronary arteries which supply the *myocardium* (the heart muscles). If these vessels become narrow due to fatty deposits or cholesterol, this will reduce the blood flow to the heart muscle, causing lack of oxygen (*ischaemia*) when exercising. This in turn could lead to a heart attack, also called a coronary attack.

Heartbeat

Most muscles will contract as a result of impulses reaching them from nerves. The heart is a muscle which beats rhythmically from impulses within its structure. It has special fibres imbedded in the wall of the right atrium called the *sinoatrial node* or, more

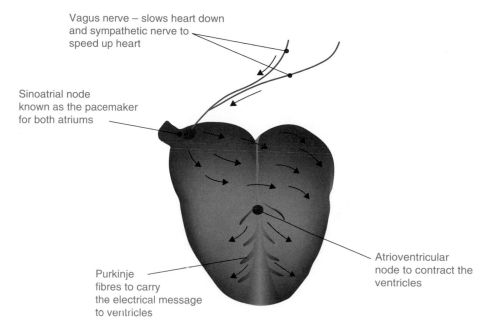

Vagus nerve – slows heart down
and sympathetic nerve to
speed up heart

Sinoatrial node
known as the pacemaker
for both atriums

Atrioventricular
node to contract the
ventricles

Purkinje
fibres to carry
the electrical message
to ventricles

Fig. 3.4 Electrical activity during contraction of the heart (pumping). The rhythm for this is provided by the pacemaker.

commonly, the *pacemaker* (Fig. 3.4). This area responds to chemicals like adrenaline or the nervous system command to increase the heart rate in situations of fear, flight or fight.

The electrical message from the pacemaker passes to the right and left atrium, causing them to contract in unison. The impulse then arrives at the atrioventricular node, before passing along special conducting tissue pathways called the *bundles of His*. These fibres lead to the smaller bundles of conducting tissues called *Purkinje fibres*, which cause contraction of the ventricles.

If the pacemaker region of the heart is malfunctioning, the heart rate may fall and not increase with exercise. An animal with this condition will have a slow heart rate with poor exercise tolerance and may faint. Heart rates vary between species (Table 3.1).

Heart sounds

There are two sounds:

Lub–Dub

The first sound, Lub, is produced by the closure of the right and left atrioventricular valves, as the ventricles begin to contract.

When the valves at the base of the aorta and pulmonary artery (semilunar valves) snap shut at the end of the ventricle contraction, then the second sound, Dub, is produced.

Table 3.1 Comparison of heart rate between species. Source: Adapted from http://www.peteducation.com/article.cfm?c=16+2160&aid=2951, accessed 13 March 2014. Reproduced with permission of Foster and Smith, Inc.

Heart rate comparison (beats/minute)		
Organism	Average rate	Normal range
Human	70	58–104
Cat	120	110–140
Cow	65	60–70
Dog	115	100–130
Guinea pig	280	260–400
Hamster	450	300–600
Horse	44	23–70
Rabbit	205	123–304
Rat	328	261–600

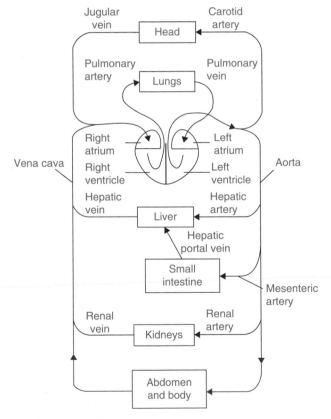

Fig. 3.5 Heart and circulation flow.

If blood within the chest is flowing unevenly or turbulently, a murmur may be detected. This sounds like Lub–woosh. The heart and flow of circulation can be seen in Figure 3.5.

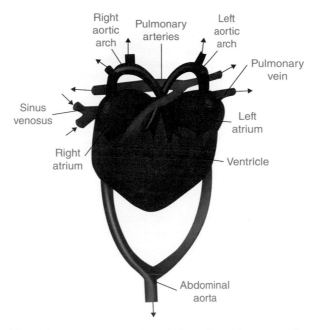

Right
aortic
arch

Pulmonary
arteries

Left
aortic
arch

Pulmonary
vein

Sinus
venosus

Left
atrium

Right
atrium

Ventricle

Abdominal
aorta

Fig. 3.6 Amphibian heart. Source: Adapted from http://www.peteducation.com/article.cfm?c=16+2160&aid=2951, accessed 13 March 2014. Reproduced with permission of Foster and Smith, Inc.

Heart structure of non-mammalian species

Avian species have a heart with four chambers like mammals. Their hearts tend to be proportionally larger than that of a mammal, possibly due to the demands that flight makes on the body. The heart of a bird also tends to pump more blood than that of a mammal of a similar size.

Reptilian species (except for crocodile species) have a heart with three chambers. The atria are separate, but the ventricles are only partially separated which means that oxygenated and deoxygenated blood mix in the heart. Reptile hearts also possess two aortas. Reptiles can exist with a three-chambered heart that is less muscular than a mammalian heart due to being ectothermic animals. It is important to note that heart structure can vary between reptile species, and this is an ongoing area of scientific investigation.

Amphibian species also have a heart with three chambers (Fig. 3.6). Heart rate in amphibians and reptiles is affected by temperature.

Fish have a heart with two chambers – one atrium and one ventricle which are separated by a simple valve. Blood is pumped from the ventricle to the gills where the blood is oxygenated (Fig. 3.7). The blood is then transported to the remainder of the body before returning to the atrium. Heart rate in fish is affected by water temperature.

The respiratory system

The respiratory system is the term given to the organs of the body which allow gaseous exchange to occur between a living organism and its environment. In the case of animals, this involves taking oxygen into the body and releasing carbon

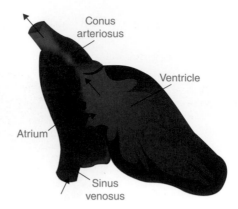

Fig. 3.7 Fish heart. Source: Adapted from http://www.peteducation.com/article.cfm?c= 16+2160&aid=2951, accessed 13 March 2014. Reproduced with permission of Foster and Smith, Inc.

dioxide as a waste product. The process of gaseous exchange in an animal is known as *respiration*.

Structures through which the oxygen and carbon dioxide must pass in a mammal are:

- *External nares* – nose
- *Turbinate bones* – scroll-shaped tubes with epithelial lining in nasal chambers
- *Nasopharynx* – back of the throat
- *Larynx* – voice box
- *Trachea* – open tube for passage of gases only
- *Bronchus* – branching of the trachea to the two sides of the chest (thorax)
- *Bronchioles* – further branching, getting smaller in diameter
- *Alveoli* – air sacs
- *Blood capillaries* of the pulmonary system
- *Tissue cells* around the body

Characteristics of respiratory surfaces

A respiratory surface is one which allows gaseous exchange to occur. They allow oxygen and carbon dioxide to be exchanged rapidly between an organism and the air which surrounds it. In order for this gaseous exchange to occur effectively and efficiently, the respiratory surface must possess certain features.

- Respiratory surfaces have a large surface area to ensure maximum contact with the inhaled air. A mammal's respiratory surface consists of millions of tiny bubble-like air sacs called *alveoli*.
- All respiratory surfaces are moist. This is necessary because oxygen and carbon dioxide can only diffuse in a solution across a respiratory surface (alveoli to blood vessel).

- A respiratory surface is very thin – only one cell thick in order for diffusion to take place.
- The inner layer of the respiratory surface is in contact with a network of capillary blood vessels to allow gas exchange to take place between the blood and gases.
- In many species of animals, a respiratory surface is usually well ventilated, in that it receives a steady flow of air. Breathing movements increase the rate of gas exchange by continually removing carbon dioxide and renewing supplies of oxygen to the tissue cells.

The role of breathing and the circulation

The respiratory and circulatory systems determine how much oxygen and carbon dioxide are present in the body at any given moment. They work together to ensure that a balance is maintained of both gases within the body. If the amount of oxygen in the blood is low and carbon dioxide high, the body responds by increasing:

- The rate and depth of breathing – ventilation rate.
- The rate at which the heart beats – cardiac frequency.
- The diameter of the arterioles serving those structures that are short of oxygen – vasodilation.

The respiratory organs of mammals

Most of the respiratory organs of animals are contained within the head and thoracic cavity – also known as thorax or chest:

- Nasal passages (found in the head)
- Pharynx and larynx
- Trachea
- Lungs
- Major blood vessels
- Lymph ducts
- Major nerves

The walls of the thorax are strengthened by the ribs (skeletal system), and caudally (towards the tail), there is a sheet of muscle called the *diaphragm*. A system of passageways leads from the mouth and nostrils into the lungs and will now be described in more detail (Fig. 3.8).

The nasal passages

The nasal passages are where air enters into the body and is warmed to body temperature. The membranes covering the nasal passages also contain the organs responsible for the sense of smell. The walls and base of the nasal passages are lined with a carpet of

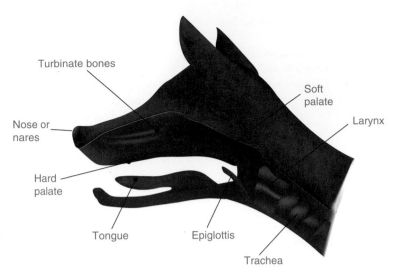

Fig. 3.8 Upper respiratory tract.

microscopic hair-like structures called *cilia*. The cilia extend down the trachea to create a surface of moving hairs beating in an upward manner. They help to expel mucus, which contains dust and micro-organisms which are held in this thickened liquid.

Air is drawn out of the nasal passages into the pharynx at the back of the mouth. From here, air is drawn into the trachea via the larynx and past the vocal cords to activate the voice of the animal.

The bronchial tree

The trachea delivers the air breathed into the body to the lungs. On reaching the lungs, the trachea branches in order to supply the lung tissue on both sides of the thorax. Each initial division feeding from the trachea into the lungs is known as a bronchus (collectively known as the bronchi) (Fig. 3.9). The bronchi will further divide many times to form a mass of fine branches called the bronchioles and so form a bronchial tree. Inflammation of the bronchi is known as bronchitis, and inflammation of the bronchioles is known as bronchiolitis.

The alveolar ducts

At the end of the bronchioles are structures called air sacs or alveoli (Fig. 3.10) where the process of gaseous exchange occurs. The alveoli are the respiratory surface of the lungs, giving lung tissue its spongy appearance. The outer surface of the alveoli is covered by a dense network of capillary blood vessels. All these capillaries originate from the pulmonary artery (deoxygenated blood) and drain into

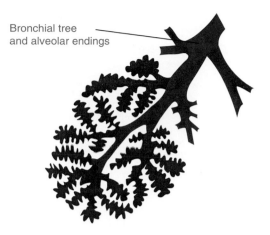

Bronchial tree
and alveolar endings

Fig. 3.9 Lung tissue.

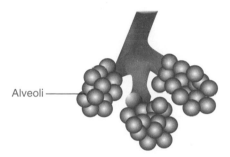

Alveoli

Fig. 3.10 Alveoli.

the pulmonary vein (oxygenated blood) to return to the left side of the heart, for pumping around the body.

Gas exchange in the lungs

Blood that enters the lungs is deoxygenated because the haemoglobin (red pigment) in its red cells has given up all its oxygen to the body tissues.

The internal diameter of the lung capillaries is actually smaller than the diameter of the red cells which pass through them. The red cells therefore are squeezed out of shape as they are forced through the lungs by blood pressure and the speed at which they move is considerably reduced by the resulting friction. This increases the rate of oxygen absorption in two ways:

(1)   As the red cells squeeze through the narrow capillaries, they expose more surface area to the capillary walls, through which oxygen is diffusing and absorbed.

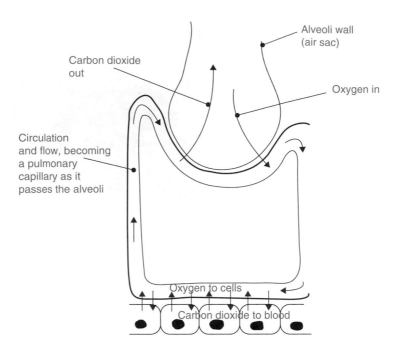

Fig. 3.11   Gas exchange between the alveoli and the blood and between the blood and body cells.

(2)   Their slow rate of progress increases the time available for oxygen to diffuse into the vessels and combine with haemoglobin.

The continuous removal of oxygen as fast as it diffuses into the lung capillaries and the continuous arrival of oxygen in the alveoli owing to breathing movements mean that there is always a higher concentration of oxygen molecules in the alveoli than in the blood. As a result of this, carbon dioxide is exchanged (Fig. 3.11).

Breathing: Ventilation of the lungs

The thorax or pleural cavity is completely airtight and contains a partial vacuum. Its internal pressure is always less than the atmospheric pressure outside the body. The lungs are open to the atmosphere through the trachea, and so there is always a higher pressure in the lungs than in the thorax or pleural cavity which surrounds them. This pressure difference is extremely important for two reasons:

(1)   The higher pressure in the lungs in relation to the pleural cavity around them stretches the thin elastic alveoli walls so that the lungs as a whole almost fill the thorax on inspiration.

(2)   Since this pressure difference is maintained during breathing movements, when the thoracic cavity increases in size (inspiration), the lungs inflate to fill the extra space available.

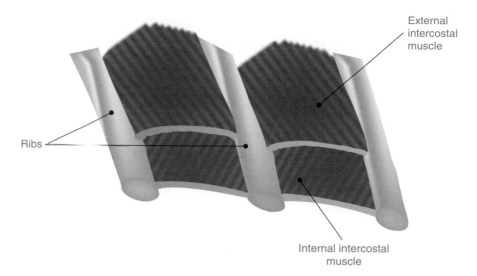

External
intercostal
muscle

Ribs

Internal intercostal
muscle

Fig. 3.12   Intercostal muscles and ribs for breathing.

At normal atmospheric pressure, the previous process could not happen, hence the need for negative pressure in the thorax.

The muscles which bring about these volume changes are:

- *The diaphragm* – a dome-shaped sheet of muscle which separates the thorax from the abdomen.
- *The intercostal muscles* – both internal and external, which cross the gap between each rib and pull the ribs outwards on inspiration (Fig. 3.12).

Diaphragm

Immediately before inspiration, the diaphragm is dome shaped and its muscle relaxed. Inspiration takes place when the diaphragm muscle contracts, making the muscle sheet a flatter shape.

Ribs

At the same time, contraction occurs in the external intercostal muscles between each rib. This increases the size of the rib cage, leading to an increase in lung volume:

- *Inspiration* – the movement of the diaphragm and external intercostal muscles, causing the ribs to move visibly outwards.
- *Expiration* – or breathing out is when the diaphragm and external intercostal muscles relax. This reduces the size of the thorax and the ribs move inwards to the resting position.

Air can be forced out of the lungs by contraction of the internal intercostal muscles, but expiration tends to be passive, simply allowing these structures to fall back into the resting position.

Respiration

The word 'respiration' is derived from the Latin *respirare* which means 'to breathe'. At first, this term referred to the breathing movements which cause air to be drawn into and pushed out of the lungs, but now, when defined with strict accuracy, respiration means something entirely different.

The modern definition of respiration

Respiration is now described as the processes which lead to, and include, the chemical breakdown of materials to provide energy for life. These processes occur inside the living cells of every type of organism and cause the release of energy from food which is essential for life.

Cells cannot use energy as soon as it is released from respiration. This energy is first used to build up a temporary energy store, which takes the form of a chemical called *adenosine triphosphate* or ATP for short. Think of ATP as 'packets' of energy used to transfer energy from the chemical reactions which release it to the body processes which use it. Respiration fills these ATP packets with energy, and they are 'emptied' when energy is needed anywhere in the body.

There are four main advantages to the ATP energy transfer system:

(1)   ATP takes up some energy which would otherwise be lost as heat during the breakdown of glucose by respiratory enzymes.
(2)   Energy is released from ATP the instant it is required without cells having to go through the many different reactions of respiration, allowing for sudden bursts of energy.
(3)   ATP delivers energy in precise amounts.
(4)   Energy can be delivered from ATP to other chemicals without energy loss, for example, from sources of sugars, fats or proteins.

The release of energy at the cellular level is known as the *Krebs cycle*.

Respiratory system in birds

Respiration in birds is much different than in mammals, mainly due to the fact that the respiratory system in birds has additional structures (Fig. 3.13):

- An organ known as the syrinx replaces the voice box. Birds do have a larynx, but it is not used for making sounds.
- As well as lungs, birds have additional unique structures called air sacs. There can be seven or nine air sacs, depending on the species of bird. The air sacs are located throughout the body cavity of the bird. The cervical air sacs are not present in some species.
- The air sacs in a bird replace the diaphragm. Pressure changes in the air sacs cause air to flow through the respiratory system of the bird. Muscular contractions in the chest area cause the sternum to be pushed put, and so air enters the respiratory system. Further muscle contraction causes air to be exhaled from the bird. It is therefore important not to hold a bird too tightly during handling; otherwise, respiration will be affected.

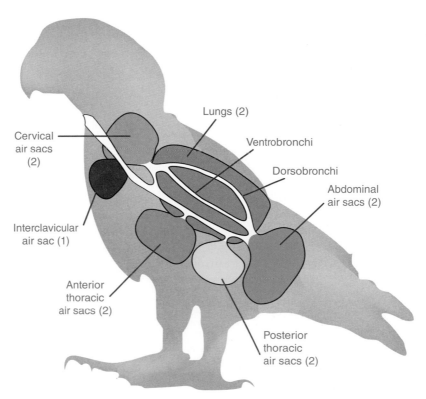

Fig. 3.13   Respiratory system of a bird. Source: Adapted from http://www.peteducation.com/
article.cfm?c=15+1829&aid=2721, accessed 13 March 2014. Reproduced with permission of
Foster and Smith, Inc.

- Gas exchange occurs in the air capillaries rather than in the alveoli.
- A bird's respiratory system is more efficient than a mammal's as more oxygen is
  released and exchanged with each breath which is beneficial to sustain flight.

Respiratory system in reptiles

The structure of the respiratory system in reptiles is similar to that in mammals, but the
mechanics of the process differ between different reptile groups. Some groups have a diaphragm; some groups don't. Some draw air into their body through the movement of their
limbs, but others have additional processes to aid breathing. Some hold their breath while
locomotion occurs, but others do not. Further research is occurring in this area of study.

Respiratory system in amphibians

Gaseous exchange can occur in amphibians in three different ways:

- Through the lungs
- Through the gills
- Through the skin

Structurally, most amphibians do not have a diaphragm. Gas exchange does not
occur through alveoli as their lungs are similar to the air sacs of birds. Amphibians

do not have a regular respiratory rate; they tend to breathe as and when they need more oxygen.

Amphibian skin allows water through as it is very thin. As water is absorbed through, then so is oxygen. During their larval stage, amphibians acquire oxygen through their gills.

Respiratory system in fish

Respiration in fish is achieved via their gills. Gills contain gill filaments in order to increase the surface area for gas exchange. A good capillary supply serves the gills and allows the efficient absorption of oxygen into the bloodstream. The gills are kept moist (as needed in a respiratory surface) by the water that surrounds the fish.

Bony fish possess an additional structure known as the operculum which protects the gills. As water is taken into the mouth of the fish, the fish moves it mouth in order to pump water through the gills, and so oxygen dissolved in the water is absorbed across the gills into the bloodstream of the fish.

Carbon dioxide is also released through the gills.

The digestive system

An animal is able to make full use of the food it eats after the following events have taken place, through the digestive tract (Fig. 3.14):

- Food is first torn up into pieces small enough to swallow (*mastication*).
- Food enters the alimentary canal mixed with digestive enzymes to further break down the food into simple water-soluble chemicals – the process of *digestion*. It takes place outside the cells of the body.

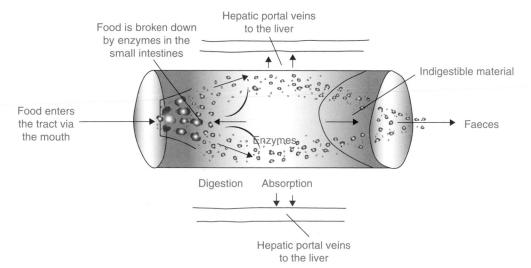

Fig. 3.14 Digestive tract – events.

- The soluble food then passes through the walls of the gut into the bloodstream. This is called *absorption*.
- Blood then transports the digested, soluble food to all parts of the body. The food enters cells and is transformed into substances which take part in the body's metabolism. This is called *assimilation*.
- Any solid substances in food which cannot be digested, like fibre, are expelled from the body as faecal matter or faeces.

Foods

Most foods which animals eat cannot be used by their bodies in the original form for two main reasons:

(1) Most foods are insoluble and so cannot pass through cell membranes into cells.
(2) Most foods are chemically different from the substances that make up body tissues. They must therefore be processed before the body can use them by the use of enzymes.

Digestive enzymes

All enzymes, whether digestive or belonging to another body system, are *catalysts*. They speed up chemical reactions which would otherwise proceed very slowly. Digestive enzymes are only one example of the many types of enzymes which exist in living animals. The reactions which these enzymes speed up involve splitting complicated molecules into simpler ones (Table 3.2).

It is thought that the enzyme combines briefly with molecules of food, and while in this state, the food undergoes a rapid chemical change in which its molecules are split apart into chemically simpler substances. These substances separate from the enzyme, leaving it immediately available for another identical reaction. Enzymes are not used up in the reactions which they control but are used countless times in rapid succession.

Table 3.2 Enzymes of the digestive tract.

Secretion	Source	Site of action	Enzyme	Acting on
Saliva	Salivary gland	Mouth	Water and mucus	All foods
Gastric juice	Stomach	Stomach	Gastrin, pepsin	Protein
Bile	Liver	Duodenum	Bile salt	Fats
Pancreatic juice	Pancreas	Duodenum*	Amylase	Starch
			Trypsin	Protein
			Lipase	Fats
Intestinal juice	Intestine wall	Small intestine	Amylase	Starch

*The cells in the duodenum release the hormone enterokinase, which activates the pancreatic enzymes only when they reach the small intestines. Otherwise, they would damage or digest the pancreas.

Comparative digestive anatomy

The digestive tract or alimentary canal is simply a continuous tube, with different regions along its length performing different functions.

Anatomically, different species of mammals are grouped according to their digestive anatomy (Figs. 3.15 and 3.16):

- Ruminants or polygastric animals (cattle and sheep)
- Simple-stomached animals (e.g. dog, cat and humans)
- Avian (all birds)
- Monogastric herbivores (the horse)

Other definitions may refer to the type of food eaten:

- Carnivores – meat eating
- Omnivores – eat both meat and plant matter
- Herbivores – plant eating

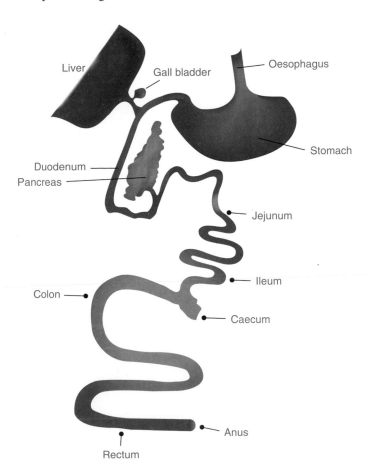

Fig. 3.15 Dog and cat digestive anatomy.

- Grainivores – grain eating
- Piscivore – fish eating
- Frugivore – fruit eating

The control of digestion of food is both voluntary and involuntary:

- Voluntary
  - (i)   Ingestion – placing in mouth
  - (ii)   Chewing
  - (iii) Swallowing (deglutition)
  - (iv)   Control of anal sphincter – the muscle controlling the opening and closing of the anus
- Involuntary
  - (i)   Opening and closing of sphincters
  - (ii)   Peristaltic movement (a ripple or wave of muscle) squeezing the food through the gut
  - (iii) Release of digestive enzymes

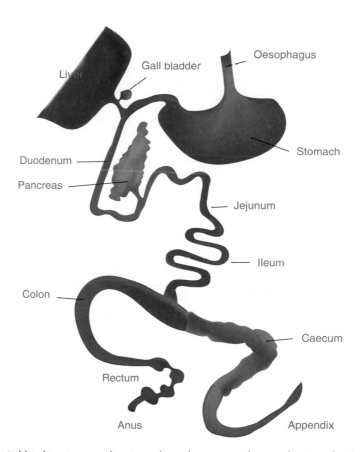

Fig. 3.16   Rabbit digestive tract showing enlarged caecum and appendix. New food is mixed with caecal (soft) pellets, which are eaten by the rabbit from its own anus (coprophagia).

Digestive tract of the dog and cat

- Mouth
- Pharynx
- Oesophagus
- Stomach
- Small intestines
  - Duodenum
  - Jejunum
  - Ileum
- Large intestines
  - Caecum
  - Ascending colon
  - Transverse colon
  - Descending colon
- Rectum
- Anal canal

The mouth

The mouth is also called the oral or buccal cavity and contains the tongue, teeth and salivary glands. The teeth are responsible for grinding, crushing or tearing up the food, and with the aid of the tongue and saliva, the food is mixed. The structure of a basic tooth is shown in Fig. 3.17. Saliva is supplied from four glands located around the face.

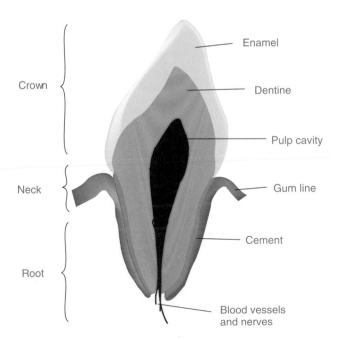

Crown

Neck

Root

Enamel

Dentine

Pulp cavity

Gum line

Cement

Blood vessels and nerves

Fig. 3.17 Structure of the basic tooth.

Saliva is usually present in the mouth, but its flow is increased by the sight and smell of food. This effect is known as a *gustatory response*. Saliva is made of water with about 1% of it being mucus, electrolytes (salts) and enzymes. The mucus acts as a lubricant and helps in the swallowing of dry food.

The tongue also helps to move the lump of food, known as a *bolus*. The tongue is a mass of striated muscle fibres. It is a sensitive structure with some of the taste buds located on its surface. The tongue has another function, especially in the cat, which is that of grooming.

Figure 3.18 shows the variation in skulls and dentition in different species.

Common to the digestive and respiratory systems is the *pharynx area*. There are lymphoid areas in the mucous membrane of this area called *tonsils*.

The processes of digestion are shown in Fig. 3.19.

The oesophagus

Pharyngeal muscles move the food bolus into the oesophagus, which is a simple tube. Swallowing or deglutition is now complete. No digestive enzymes are secreted here, but oesophageal cells produce mucus to lubricate the process of peristalsis, the wave-like contraction and relaxation which will propel the food along the tract (Fig. 3.20). These contractions are stimulated by the presence of food.

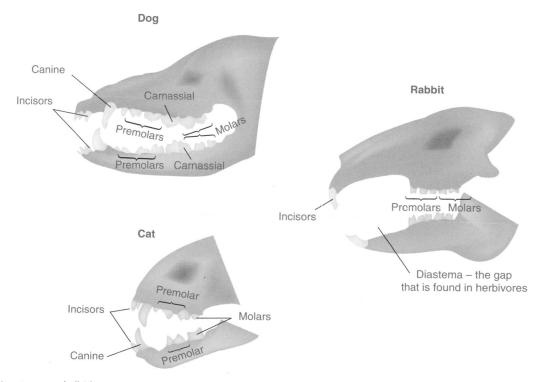

Fig. 3.18   Skull/dentition variation.

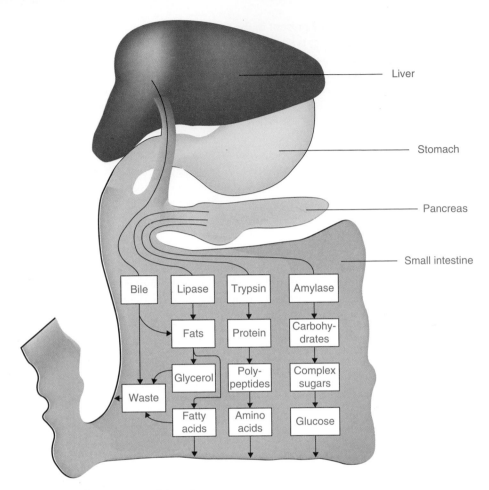

Fig. 3.19 The processes of digestion.

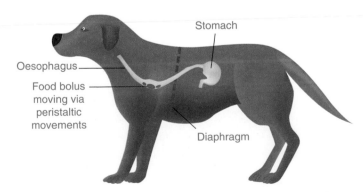

Fig. 3.20 Oesophagus and stomach showing food being moved by peristalsis.

Dental formula

Dental formula is used to indicate the different types of teeth in the mouth and also the number that should be present at a certain stage of life in a species.

Dog   Deciduous or milk teeth $- I\frac{3}{3}C\frac{1}{1}PM\frac{3}{3} = $ Total 28

Permanent or adult teeth $- I\frac{3}{3}C\frac{1}{1}PM\frac{4}{4}M\frac{2}{3} = $ Total 42

Cat   Deciduous $- I\frac{3}{3}C\frac{1}{1}PM\frac{3}{2} = $ Total 26

Permanent $- I\frac{3}{3}C\frac{1}{1}PM\frac{3}{2}M\frac{1}{1} = $ Total 30

Rabbit   Open rooted $- I\frac{2}{1}C\frac{0}{0}PM\frac{3}{2}M\frac{3}{3} = $ Total 14

The stomach

The oesophagus enters the stomach via a ring of muscle called the *cardiac sphincter,* a structure which adapts itself to the quantity of food eaten. Some digestion occurs here and the stomach acts as a temporary reservoir. The gastric juices, which contain enzymes and hydrochloric acid, start breaking up the food. The well-mixed and partially digested food, now called *chyme,* is now moved through the sphincter at the stomach exit, called the *pylorus,* and onto the first section of the small intestine.

The small intestines

The small intestines are so-called because of their narrow bore, not their length. Enzyme digestion is completed in the small intestines:

- Protein is converted to amino acids
- Fat is converted to fatty acids
- Carbohydrates are converted to simple sugars

The chyme is mixed with more enzymes in the first section of the small intestines, the *duodenum.* Some will originate from the duodenum, and others from the *pancreas* (its *exocrine* function). The liver also secretes a digestive fluid into the duodenum via the gall bladder; this fluid is ducted into the small intestine to reduce the size of fatty acid molecules and is called *bile.* Bile helps by emulsifying fats and will neutralize the acid fluids from the stomach because it is alkaline.

The second section of the small intestines, called the *jejunum,* continues the mixing and exposing of the chyme to the fluids that reduce it sufficiently for absorption.

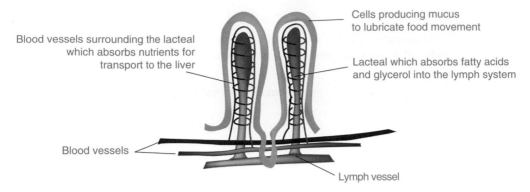

Cells producing mucus
to lubricate food movement

Blood vessels surrounding the lacteal
which absorbs nutrients for
transport to the liver

Lacteal which absorbs fatty acids
and glycerol into the lymph system

Blood vessels

Lymph vessel

Fig. 3.21   The villi.

The third section of the small intestines is the *ileum*, where the final absorption is completed.

Digestion and absorption are improved by the enormous surface area in the small intestine. Features of this area include:

- The great length of the intestines
- The presence of folds of tissue, increasing the surface area
- The arrangement of fingerlike projections called *villi*
- The great number of these villi on the surface of the small intestine, particularly in the final area, the ileum, for maximum absorption

Absorption. This takes place via the villi (Fig. 3.21). They contain smooth muscle which allows them to contract and expand. This action brings them into contact with the newly digested food. Simple sugars (mainly glucose) and amino acids are absorbed, by a combination of diffusion and active transport, across the epithelial lining of the villi into the waiting capillaries beneath. These capillaries drain into the hepatic portal vein which leads to the liver.

Fat is dealt with differently. The fatty acids and glycerol are absorbed into the columnar epithelial cells lining the villi and are pushed into the lymph vessels of the villi as a white emulsion of tiny globules of fat. These globules give the lymph vessels a milky appearance, for which they are known as *lacteals*. The lymph system opens finally into the veins in the thorax and empties via the thoracic duct into the vena cava near the heart.

Mineral salts, vitamins and water are also absorbed in the small intestine.

The large intestines

This section of intestines is a wider tube and contains no villi. Food materials which are of no value or cannot be broken down to absorbable size are passed from the small to the large intestine through the *ileocaecal valve*. The large intestine in the dog and cat is relatively short in length. Its main purpose is to absorb salt and water. The walls of the colon (large intestine) are much folded for this purpose. By the time the materials reach the rectum, indigestible food is in a semisolid condition ready to be voided through the anus as faeces.

The first part of the large intestines is called the *caecum*. It is a blind-ended sac which has no function in carnivores but is enlarged in herbivores as a site of bacterial breakdown of vegetable food matter.

The colon is divided into three sections:

- Ascending
- Transverse
- Descending

The colon terminates in the rectum area, where waste products are held before excretion as faecal material.

The last part of the tract is closed by sphincter muscles and is known as the anal canal, over which the animal has control via skeletal muscle (voluntary muscle). Defaecation involves relaxation of the anal sphincter, but diarrhoea or illness may override this control. Diarrhoea is defined as the frequent evacuation of watery faeces. If defaecation is delayed too long, constipation may result.

Consistent with its functions of water absorption and faecal movement, the large intestine is lined with a mucous-secreting surface. This assists in the movement of materials by a lubricating action. The mucus prevents the total drying out of the faeces, which might then damage the lining.

The following is a brief summary of digestion and absorption of the main food constituents:

- *Proteins* – come from muscle meat, egg or vegetable proteins like soya bean. These are broken down in the stomach and small intestines to become amino acids and absorbed into the bloodstream for transport to the liver, where they are processed.
- *Carbohydrates* – are found as cereals like biscuit potatoes or pasta. They are broken down into simple sugars (*glucose*) and absorbed into the bloodstream for transport to the liver where they may be stored as *glycogen*. When required by the body for energy, glycogen can be turned back into glucose.
- *Fats* – are found as animal fat or vegetable oils and are broken down into fatty acids and glycerols by bile and enzymes in the small intestines. Most will enter the lacteals in the villi to travel via the lymph system, finally reaching the bloodstream for use or storage.

The liver

The liver is the largest organ of the body, situated immediately caudal to the diaphragm in the abdomen. About 75% of the liver's blood supply comes from the hepatic portal system of vessels (Fig. 3.22). This ensures that the products of digestion are absorbed into the bloodstream and travel to the liver for processing, before moving on either to storage or to be used in another way. The remaining 25% of blood to the liver arrives via the hepatic artery.

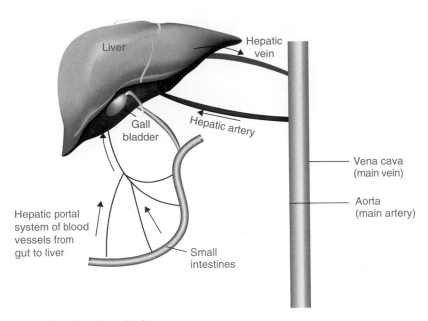

Fig. 3.22 Blood supply to the liver.

The special cells that make up the liver are called *hepatocytes*. The liver is a very complex chemical factory which produces materials for use within the body from the products of digestion which come directly to it from the gut.

Functions of the liver It is thought that the liver performs over 500 functions. The main functions are as follows:

- Regulation of sugar which has four possible fates:
  - used as an energy source (Krebs cycle)
  - stored as glycogen in the liver
  - converted to fat and stored around the body
  - passed directly into the circulation
- Regulation of lipids (fats)
- Regulation of amino acids and proteins
- Heat production
- Bile production
- Formation of cholesterol
- Elimination of sex hormones
- Storage and filtration of blood
- Elimination of haemoglobin from exhausted red blood cells
- Formation of urea to be passed on to the kidneys for removal from the body
- Creation of plasma proteins (synthesis)
- Storage of vitamins A, D and B_{12} and minerals like iron and copper

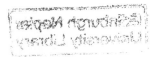

The pancreas

The pancreas is a large grey-pink gland, which lies in the abdomen close to the stomach and the duodenum section of the small intestine. It is made up of two parts which are joined together, giving the pancreas its boomerang shape.

There are two types of tissue present within the gland, and these have very different functions:

- *Exocrine tissue* – produces digestive enzymes
- *Endocrine tissue* – produces hormones like insulin to help in controlling sugar in the body.

The urinary system

This system has several functions, but its main one is that of excretion and removal of waste products from the body. Wastes are toxic if allowed to accumulate, so this removal of harmful materials, which are the end products of metabolism, is essential and continuous.

The mammalian urinary tract consists of:

- Two kidneys
- Two ureters
- One bladder
- One urethra

Functions of the urinary system include:

- loss or conservation of body water
- excretion of unwanted substances or those in excess to requirements
- storage of products before their removal from the body
- endocrine organ producing hormones.

The kidneys

The kidneys are bean shaped and situated one on each side of the abdomen (Fig. 3.23). Each contains specialized cells which filter out materials which must be removed from the body and conserve those which the body needs. These cells are called the *nephrons*, from which we get the term *nephritis*, meaning inflammation of the kidney nephron cells.

The blood supply to the kidneys is via the renal artery directly from the aorta and drains away from the kidney via the renal vein directly into the vena cava.

The nephron

This is the special cell of the urinary system. The structure is as follows (Fig. 3.24):

- *Glomerulus* – a network or knot of artery from branches of the renal artery in the cortex section of the kidney.

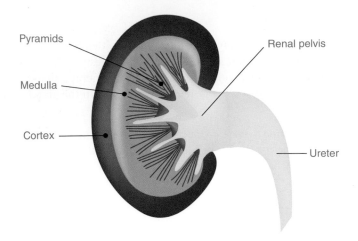

Fig. 3.23 The kidney.

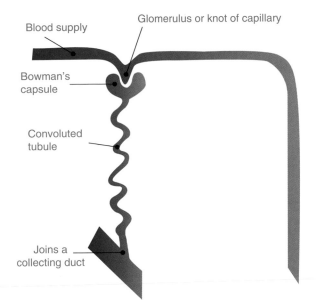

Fig. 3.24 The nephron.

- *Bowman's capsule* – the cup-shaped part of the nephron at the start of the tubule. It is into this that the glomerulus fits and contacts, resulting in the start of blood filtration and the removal of urea and other nitrogenous wastes.
- *Proximal tubule* – the start of the long tube through which the filtered substances will pass.
- *Loop of Henle and distal tubule* – this is where, on instruction from hormones, the nephron conserves water, salts and sugars or, if the body has an excess, it is instructed to add the excess to the forming urine for removal from the body.

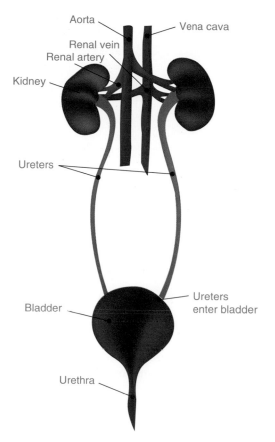

Aorta

Vena cava

Renal vein

Renal artery

Kidney

Ureters

Bladder

Ureters
enter bladder

Urethra

Fig. 3.25 The urinary system.

The distal tubule joins a collecting duct which directs the urine to the pelvis region of the kidney, where all nephrons drain, then along the ureter to the bladder for temporary storage. When the bladder is full, the animal receives this information from the brain and relaxes the sphincter muscle from the bladder to the urethra and the outside (Fig. 3.25). The act of passing urine is called *micturition*.

The nervous system

The nervous system provides the quickest means of communication within the body. Information is received both from outside the animal (the environment) and from inside the animal's body. The response to information received has to be co-ordinated in order for the body systems to unite in their response to produce the desired effect.

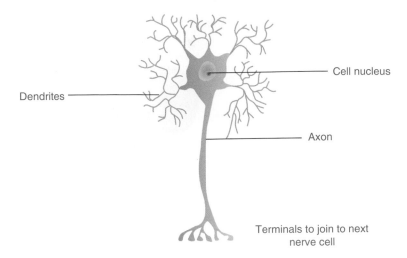

Cell nucleus

Dendrites

Axon

Terminals to join to next
nerve cell

Fig. 3.26 Nerve cell – the neurone.

Messages to the body are carried in two ways:

(1) *Electrical* – these are impulses which travel along the nerves and give fast response
to a situation or stimulus (nervous system). The electrical messages stimulate
movement of muscles:
  (a) cardiac – the heart
  (b) skeletal – bones and joints
  (c) involuntary – organs and tissues.
(2) *Chemical* – these are hormones which, once released into the bloodstream, will
travel more slowly to their target organ. The body response is seen after a period of
time (endocrine system).

Body co-ordination by nervous system tissue is conducted by the nerve cells, the
neurones (Fig. 3.26), together with various forms of supporting tissue in which they
are embedded. These cells are the basic functional unit of the nervous system and are
found in bundles, called *nerves*.
  There are four types of neurone:

(1) *Sensory* – those attached to the senses, like sight, hearing, taste, smell and touch.
These carry messages about information outside the body to the brain.
(2) *Relay* – information or messages between neurones.
(3) *Motor* – these link up to relay neurones and with muscle or gland cells in order to
deliver messages from the central nervous system (brain and spinal cord) to initiate
an action. This may be the release of more hormones or the movement of a
muscle.
(4) *Network* – these link the cell branches in order to keep the information and action
by the brain and spinal cord networked like a computer.

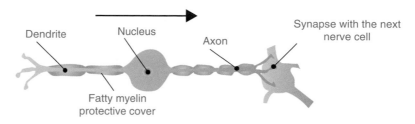

Fig. 3.27 Nerve cell and direction of electrical impulse.

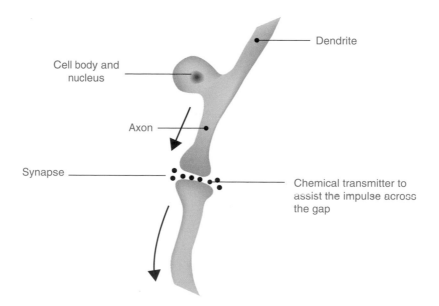

Fig. 3.28 A synapse – the junction between two or more neurones.

The shape of the nerve cell will vary to suit the tissue into which it links, but the basic components remain the same:

- A cell body containing the nucleus.
- Cell processes which lead to and from the cell body (Fig. 3.27):
  (a) the *axon* – which carries the impulses away from the cell body
  (b) the *dendrite* – which carries impulses towards the cell body.

The property of a nerve cell is that its cell membrane is electrically charged by the action of *ions* (salts or electrolytes) such as potassium or sodium. Although the voltage carried is small, when discharged along the length of nerves, it allows the system to act as a high-speed electrical signalling system. After the signal, the membrane is recharged and returns to a resting position, awaiting the next signal.

The junction between two or more neurones is called a *synapse* (Fig. 3.28). Electrical impulses cannot pass across this gap, so communication is dependent upon a chemical transmitter substance – a *neurotransmitter*. This substance will connect two neurones

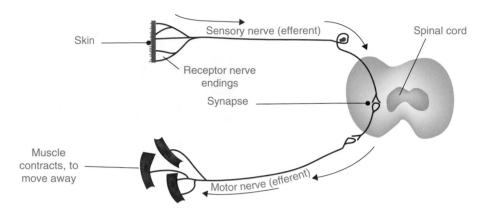

Fig. 3.29 Reflex arc.

for less than 1 millisecond, allowing the impulse to pass on. The chemical is then destroyed by another substance and recreated again before each future impulse.

Reflex action or arc (Fig. 3.29)

This refers to an automatic and very rapid response to a potentially harmful stimulus which is usually external to the body. It is a survival response.

The structural basis of reflex action is the *reflex arc*, which represents the series of units of nerve tissue through which impulses have to pass in order to bring about a reflex response. The sensory tissues receiving the information are called *receptors* and may be scattered sensory cells in the skin or special sense receptors like the eye or ear. Their stimulation results in impulses being generated in sensory (*afferent*) neurones located in the peripheral nerves (on or near the body surface). These afferent neurones take the impulse to the central nervous system (only to the spinal cord) where a connection nerve in the cord connects to a motor (*efferent*) neurone. This will take the impulse or message to an effector tissue like a gland or to a muscle for the desired effect – survival.

The common example used is touching a hot surface, when the reflex arc ensures that the animal suffers minimal harm as the foot is speedily withdrawn from the danger.

Central nervous system

The central nervous system comprises the brain and the spinal cord.

The brain

The general function of the brain is to co-ordinate the body's activities. It receives all sensory information and processes it for:

- Immediate use – reflex arc.
- Later use – storing it in memory, passing orders via neurones and hormones and constantly monitoring the internal body systems for any change.

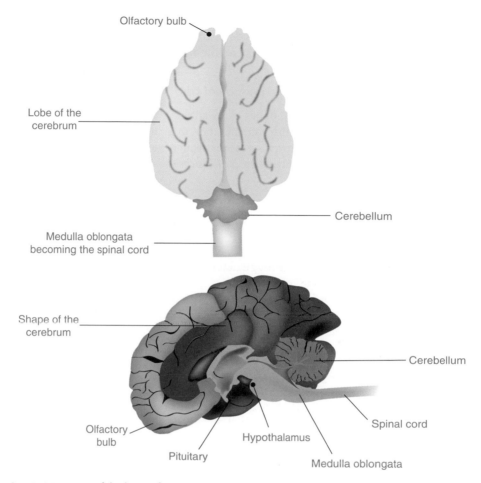

Fig. 3.30 Parts of the brain, from two views.

The brain is divided into three parts (Fig. 3.30):

- *Forebrain* – cerebrum, divided into two areas called the cerebral hemispheres (including the hypothalamus) and involved with voluntary movement and the senses.
- *Midbrain* – involved with sight, hearing, muscle control and body position.
- *Hindbrain* – the cerebellum, the pons and the medulla oblongata. It is involved with complicated movements of the body, control of the circulation and respiration and awareness of surroundings.

The spinal cord

The cord extends from the base of the skull to the lumbar/sacral region of the spine, over the pelvis. It is a continuation of the hindbrain and medulla oblongata. The cord is protected by the *vertebrae* and the *meninges*. The canal, which runs through each vertebra, houses the spinal cord.

The cord divides into many branching spinal nerves. This continues first inside the vertebrae, then on the outside of the coccygeal vertebrae as the *cauda equina* (resembling a horse's tail), to supply motor and sensory nerves to the tip of the animal's tail.

Protection of the brain and spinal cord

- *Bones* – skull and bones of the spine.
- *Meninges* – the three membranes, in turn separated by the cerebrospinal fluid.
- *Blood–brain barrier* – a mechanism located in a continuous layer of endothelial cells which allows only useful substances to enter the brain.

Meninges

The three protective membranes covering the brain and spinal cord are:

- *Dura mater* – the tough outer membrane, in contact with the bone of the skull and the vertebrae.
- *Arachnoid mater* – a fine network of collagen and elastic fibres, next to the dura mater.
- *Pia mater* – the membrane in contact with the brain and spinal cord tissue surface.

Peripheral nervous system

The peripheral nervous system receives the information from the animal's surrounding environment and transfers it to the central nervous system where a response is co-ordinated.

The peripheral nervous system is comprised of the voluntary and involuntary nervous systems.

Voluntary nervous system

- Paired spinal nerves containing both sensory and motor fibres, forming a mixed spinal nerve.
- Twelve cranial nerves. These are mixed nerves and can contain motor and sensory, voluntary and autonomic fibres (Table 3.3).

Involuntary or autonomic nervous system

- Sympathetic nervous system
- Parasympathetic nervous system

The involuntary or autonomic nervous system is not under conscious control and is involved with the regulation of body functions. It is divided into two parts, distinguished by their function and by the chemical transmitters (neurotransmitters) used at the synapse between nerve cells (Table 3.4).

Table 3.3 The 12 cranial nerves.

Number	Name	Type	Function
I	Olfactory	Sensory	Smell
II	Optic	Sensory	Vision, pupil light response
III	Oculomotor	Motor	Eye movement, pupil constriction
IV	Trochlear	Motor	Eye movement
V	Trigeminal	Mixed	Mastication, touch and pain receptors
VI	Abducens	Motor	Eye movement
VII	Facial	Mixed	Salivation, facial expression, taste
VIII	Auditory/ vestibulocochlear	Sensory	Hearing, balance
IX	Glossopharyngeal	Mixed	Taste, laryngeal muscles
X	Vagus	Mixed	Vocalization, swallowing Decrease in heart rate Abdominal organs
XI	Accessory	Motor	Head movement
XII	Hypoglossal	Motor	Tongue movement

Table 3.4 Function of neurotransmitters.

Sympathetic system	Parasympathetic system
• Chemical – adrenaline	• Chemical – cholinesterase
• Prepares body for fight, fright and flight	• Stimulates salivation
• Inhibits salivation	• Assists in day-to-day function of the body
• Increases heart rate	• Decreases heart rate to normal
• Increases respiratory rate	• Decreases respiratory rate

The endocrine system

This is made up of a system of ductless glands which are sites for the production of hormones (Fig. 3.31). The hormones are discharged directly into the blood for circulation to the target organ or tissue. Hormones are sometimes referred to as chemical messengers.

The word 'endocrine' means 'internal secretion', and the organs of this system are therefore glands of internal secretion. Although the glands are sited all over the body, they influence one another and, through their interactions, are integrated into a highly co-ordinated system.

The messages from the hormones:

• Have long-lasting effects on their targets (hours to days)
• Assist in the constant adjustment of the internal body
• Arrive at their target at the speed of the circulating blood

The nervous and endocrine systems are linked. The endocrine gland that controls the functions of all the other glands in this system, the pituitary or master gland, is in the brain close to the hypothalamus.

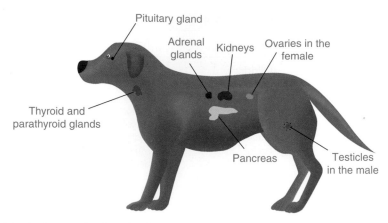

Fig. 3.31 Endocrine glands in the dog.

Endocrine glands

Pituitary gland

Controlling the other glands, body growth and the internal body, the pituitary is situated at the base of the brain. It is divided into two parts:

- The anterior pituitary
- The posterior pituitary

The *anterior* pituitary produces:

- Thyrotropic or thyroid-stimulating hormone (TSH) for production of thyroid hormone.
- Adrenocorticotropic hormone (ACTH) for control of adrenal glands and release of corticosteroids.
- Growth hormone (GH) or somatotropin which promotes the body's growth.
- Gonadotropins which influence the ovaries and testes:
  (a) follicle-stimulating hormone (FSH) promotes the ripening of the eggs in the ovaries and the secretion of oestrogen in the female. In the male, FSH assists the development of the sperm cells
  (b) luteinizing hormone (LH) stimulates ovulation and the secretion of oestrogen and progesterone in the female. In the male, it stimulates the development and release of testosterone
  (c) prolactin or lactogenic hormone develops mammary tissues during pregnancy for milk production.

The *posterior pituitary* produces:

- Antidiuretic hormone (ADH) or vasopressin, which prevents excessive loss of water from the body via the kidneys.
- Oxytocin which stimulates the release of milk and uterine contractions during parturition.

Thyroid gland

The thyroid gland regulates growth, body development and metabolism. It is located below the larynx near the trachea. It produces and secretes the thyroid hormone which regulates metabolism, growth and development.

Parathyroid glands

The parathyroid glands are situated near the thyroid gland. It produces parathyroid hormone (PTH) which regulates the calcium and phosphorus levels in the blood and bones.

Adrenal gland

The adrenal gland regulates the growth of bones, muscle development and secondary sex characteristics. These two small glands are located near the kidneys. The glands are divided into:

- *Cortex* – producing steroids, which are concerned with the regulation of sodium and potassium and the body water (fluids) balance. An example of a hormone produced here is aldosterone. Corticosteroids produced assist in the metabolism of nutrients, antibody formation and dealing with stress. Also produced here are the hormones responsible for the male and female sex characteristics.
- *Medulla* – secretes adrenaline and noradrenaline, which prepare the body for fight or flight in stressful situations.

The pancreas

The pancreas regulates the use and storage of glucose in the body and is considered a part of the digestive system. It lies close to the stomach in a loop of the small intestine (duodenum). It produces insulin for the use and storage of simple sugars from the breakdown of carbohydrates in the diet.

Pineal gland

This is a small oval gland situated near the base of the brain. It secretes melatonin, which inhibits gonad activity. The secretions may be linked to seasonal light levels, which control timing of an animal's oestrous cycle.

Gonads

Female (ovaries) and male (testes) gonads produce hormones for the functioning of the reproductive systems of each sex:

- *Ovaries* – produce some of the oestrogen hormone responsible for the secondary sex characteristics and oestrous cycles. They also produce progesterone for the preparation of the uterus in pregnancy.
- *Testes* – produce testosterone, responsible for male secondary sex characteristics.

The following organs are not endocrine glands but do produce hormones:

- *Kidney* – produces the hormone erythropoietin, which stimulates the production of red cells in active bone marrow sites.
- *Intestines* – produce hormones to promote the production of digestive enzyme compounds from organs such as the pancreas. Regulatory enzymes are also produced that control appetite.

The sense organs

Sense organs collect information from the surrounding environment, both internal and external. Each piece of information received is known as a stimulus. However, sensations are interpreted by the brain once it is fed the information via nerves. Sense organs collect information from inside and outside the body:

Inside the body

- Temperature monitored by the hypothalamus of the brain.
- Regulation of breathing by measuring the carbon dioxide levels.
- Tension of muscles or tendons which prevents over-exercise and damage.

Outside the body

- Light, dark, shape or colour becomes sight.
- Sound and changes of body position become hearing and balance.
- Airborne chemicals become smells.
- Ingested chemicals become tastes.
- Touch, heat and cold pass survival information to the brain.

The eye

This is the organ of vision (Fig. 3.32). The eye resembles a camera in at least three ways:

(1) Both focus light. In the eye, the apparatus for this consists of the transparent cornea and lens. These act like the glass lens of the camera in forming the image.
(2) This image falls on a layer of receptors called the retina which, like the film in a camera, is sensitive to light.
(3) Eyes and cameras have a mechanism called an iris diaphragm, which is an opaque disc with a hole at the centre. This increases or decreases in size to control light entering the eye.

The retina transforms light into a stream of nerve impulses which pass down the optic nerve to the brain to form a picture. The frequency and pattern of these impulses vary

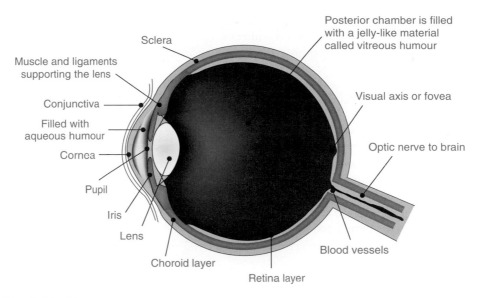

Fig. 3.32   The eye.

according to patches of colour, light and shade which make up the retinal image. The visual area of the brain interprets these impulses to form moving impressions.

Protection of the eyes

- Cavities in the skull called the *orbits* protect the eyeball with a bone and cartilage ring.
- The transparent, self-repairing skin on the eye called the conjunctiva.
- Tears keep the eyes moist; a stream of liquid from the tear glands is wiped across the eye by blinking and prevents the tissues from becoming too dry.
- The blink reflex to guard against dust and other objects which might enter the eye socket.

Nourishment and support tissues of the eye

- The eye receives oxygen via the blood vessels which enter with the optic nerve, at the back of the eye. These vessels spread out through the *choroid layer* and over the surface of the *retina*.
- The *cornea* and *lens* obtain oxygen and food by diffusion from vessels in the liquid in the front chamber of the eye – the *aqueous humour*.
- *Vitreous humour* is a jelly in the back cavity of the eye which helps to maintain the shape of the eye.
- The *iris* is the coloured part of the eye and has a round hole in its centre called the *pupil*. The iris consists of muscles which radiate out and contract to enlarge the size

of the pupil and circular muscles, which make it smaller in size. The iris regulates the amount of light reaching the retina.

- The *lens* consists of layers of transparent material arranged like the skins of an onion, which are enclosed in an elastic outer membrane. These are held in place by *suspensory ligaments*, which in turn are attached to a ring of muscle called the *ciliary muscle*.
- The retina is covered with light-sensitive receptors called *rods and cones* (due to their shape). These are buried under nerve fibres and a layer of blood capillaries which conduct the impulses to the brain. These layers are absent from the area where the clearest image is formed, the *fovea*. This area is directly opposite the lens and is the most sensitive part of the eye for colour vision.
- The retina contains an area called the *blind spot* (Fig. 3.33). It consists of blood vessels and nerve fibres leading to the optic nerve. Due to these tissues, this area is completely insensitive to light.

Fig. 3.33 Detecting the eye's blind spot.

Hold this page with the cross and spot at arm's length.

Close the left eye and stare at the cross with the right eye. Note that the black circle is still visible.

Bring the page slowly towards the face. At a certain point, the circle will disappear.

This happens when its image falls on the blind spot.

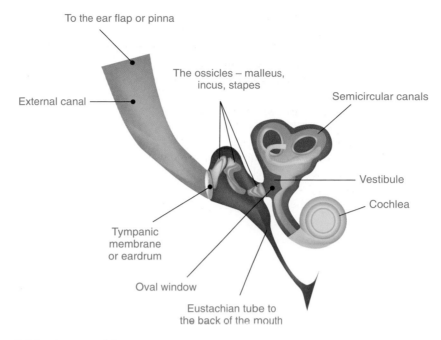

To the ear flap or pinna

The ossicles – malleus,
incus, stapes

Semicircular canals

External canal

Vestibule

Cochlea

Tympanic
membrane
or eardrum

Oval window

Eustachian tube to
the back of the mouth

Fig. 3.34 Anatomy of the ear.

The ear

The anatomy of the ear is shown in Fig. 3.34. The functions of the ear are:

- Hearing
- Detecting change in body position
- Balance

The ear is divided into three sections:

(1) *Outer* – for sound gathering.
(2) *Middle* – transmits vibrations to the oval window of the inner ear.
(3) *Inner* – receives the sound waves and passes them to the nerve that connects to the
brain for conversion into hearing.

Outer ear

This is made up of the ear flap or *pinna* and the canal. The shape of the canal will vary
between species and breeds. This part of the ear collects sound waves and directs
them into the canal, which is lined with modified sebaceous glands. These glands
produce wax, as a protective layer. The canal leads to the eardrum or *tympanic
membrane*.

Middle ear

This lies beyond the eardrum in the tympanic cavity, which is made of bone, on the ventral surface of the skull. The cavity contains three small bones called *ossicles*:

- *Malleus* – known as the hammer (contacts the eardrum)
- *Incus* – known as the anvil
- *Stapes* – known as the stirrup (contacts the oval window)

The vibrations of the eardrum (tympanic membrane) are transmitted by these bones to the *oval window*, which is the junction between the middle and inner ear.

The link between the middle ear and the throat/pharynx is the *auditory tube* (*Eustachian tube*). This tube allows air pressure to be equalized on either side of the eardrum.

Inner ear

This is situated in the temporal bone of the skull. It is here that sound vibrations are converted into nervous impulses and the inner ear is also involved in maintaining balance.

This area consists of a closed system of delicate tubes, called the *membranous labyrinth*, which contains a fluid called *endolymph*. The labyrinth is itself bathed in a separate fluid, the *perilymph*.

The labyrinth is made up of:

- The *vestibule* – a sac-like structure.
- The *semicircular canals* – these are three loops at right angles to each other. They respond to the movement of the endolymph, the angle of the head and changes in body position.
- The *cochlea* – a snail-shaped structure responsible for converting sound waves into nerve impulses which are converted in the brain to hearing.

Other senses

- *Smell* or olfaction is important for the selection of food and scenting other animals. Olfactory membranes can also receive stimuli from the mouth, so as a result, taste is sometimes actually smell. For some species, the smell is the major sense through which they detect changes in their environment, e.g. star-nosed mole.
- *Taste* or gustation arises from taste cells contained in the mucous membranes of the mouth and on the base of the tongue. Taste and smell will stimulate salivation and the digestive tract in readiness for food to be swallowed.
- *Jacobson's organ*, or the vomeronasal organ, supplements the sense of smell in receiving pheromone information about other animals. It is involved in the location of an animal on heat for reproductive purposes.

The skin

The skin is also known as the integument and is the outer protective layer of the body. The anatomy of the skin is shown in Fig. 3.35.

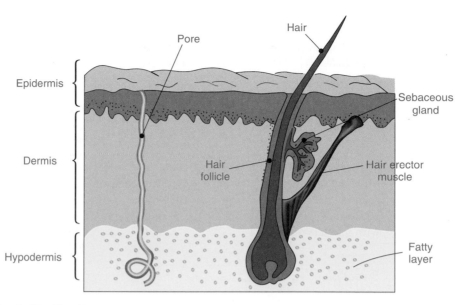

Fig. 3.35 The skin.

Function of the skin

- *Protection* – from the external environment and the controlled internal environment of the body, actively preventing:
  - (a) water loss
  - (b) absorption of toxic or harmful substances
  - (c) entry of disease-producing micro-organisms (*pathogens*).
- *Production* – of vitamin D which is required for the absorption of calcium from the intestines.
- *Sense organ* – receptor nerves throughout the skin's surface respond to:
  - (a) touch
  - (b) temperature
  - (c) pressure
  - (d) pain.
- *Storage* – of fat as adipose tissue. This is a body energy store and acts as an insulation layer to help maintain body temperature in cold weather.
- *Temperature control*
  - (a) For heat loss:
    - – vasodilation of surface blood vessels (widening of the vessel wall)
    - – sweating.
  - (b) For heat gain:
    - – vasoconstriction of blood vessels (narrowing of the vessel wall)
    - – erection of surface hair/coat/feathers to trap a layer of air for insulation
    - – a fat layer under the skin (*subcutaneous layer*).
- *Scent gland* – for communication with other animals for reproductive purposes (production of pheromones) or territorial purposes (use of the anal glands on either side of the anus).

Structure of the skin

- *Epidermis* – is the outer layer, which is hard and dry and contains no blood vessels. This layer continually looses dead cells.
- *Dermis* – is the layer below the epidermis and is a type of connective tissue containing nerves, blood vessels, glands and hair roots.
- *Hypodermis* – is the innermost layer of the skin.

Hair

This covers most of a mammal's surface area. It is made of *keratin* (a protein made by the body) and pigments for colour. It grows from the hair *follicle*, and attached to the deepest section of the hair is the smooth (involuntary) muscle called the *erector pili* muscle which is responsible for moving the hair upright. In other species, hair may be replaced with feathers or scales.

Sweat glands

Sweat or sebaceous glands produce *sebum* which will include a pheromone. Other very specialized glands in the skin include mammary glands for milk production and anal glands for scenting territory.

The skeleton

The anatomy of the skeleton is shown in Fig. 3.36a. Figure 3.36b and 3.36c shows the differences between dog and cat skeletons.

The skeleton is divided into three parts:

(1) *Axial* – skull, vertebral column (spine), ribs and sternum.
(2) *Appendicular* – the fore- and hindlimbs.
(3) *Splanchnic* – bones that develop in tissues, such as the os penis and fabellae.

Anatomical position terms

- *Proximal* – meaning 'nearer to the centre of the body' (e.g. the part of the femur bone closest to the hip joint would be called the proximal end of femur).
- *Distal* – meaning 'further from the centre of the body' (e.g. the part of the femur bone nearest to the knee or stifle would be called the distal end of femur).
- *Cranial* – descriptive term meaning 'towards or within the head'.
- *Dorsal* – the surface of the body which is on top.
- *Caudal* – a descriptive term meaning 'towards or within the tail'.
- *Medial* – a term describing something that lies nearest to the midline of the body.
- *Ventral* – any surface of the body that is facing the ground.
- *Lateral* – the sides of the body, both left and right.

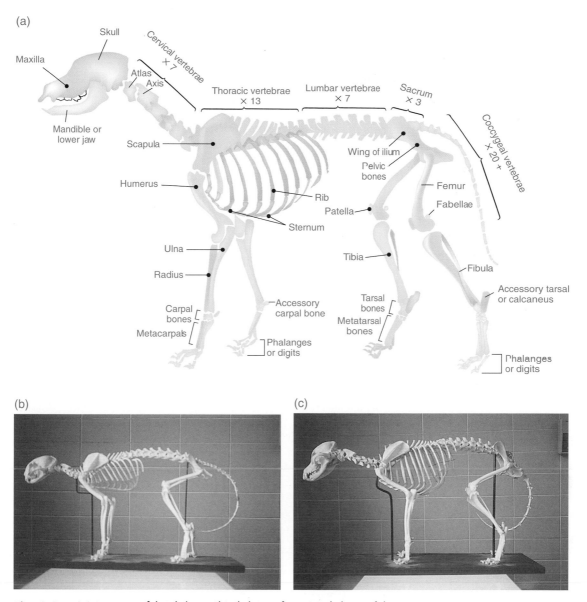

Fig. 3.36   (a) Anatomy of the skeleton. (b) Skeleton of cat. (c) Skeleton of dog.

Movements of the body

These are movements of a whole limb relative to the body:

- *Protraction* – movement of a limb towards the head (cranially).
- *Retraction* – movement of a limb towards the tail (caudally).
- *Elevation* – movement of a limb up and nearer the body (proximal to body).

- *Adduction* – movement of a limb towards the middle of the body (midline).
- *Abduction* – movement of a limb away from the middle of the body (away from the midline).

Bone structure

Bone is hard and to some extent also flexible (Fig. 3.37). The cells in bone are arranged as cylinders and in layers in order to give bone its strength. They also secrete minerals like calcium and phosphorus, which provide its rigid nature. The structure of bones provides for the maximum resistance to mechanical stresses, while maintaining the least bony mass. Bone is made of two types of cells:

- *Osteoblasts* are responsible for the secretion of material which, when mineralized, will become bone. Osteoblasts become trapped in the forming bone and are then called *osteocytes*.
- *Osteoclasts* are responsible for reabsorbing materials and therefore for the remodelling of bone.

In the general structure of long bones, there are two types of bone materials:

- *Compact* bone which will form the dense walls of the bone shaft.
- *Cancellous* or *spongy* bone which is found in the central medullary cavity. As the name suggests, this bone consists of a network and spaces all linked to each other.

The *medullary cavity* of most bones contains active or red marrow which is responsible for the production of platelets, red and white blood cells. The yellow, rather fatty-looking, material sometimes found in the medullary cavities is the inactive bone marrow.

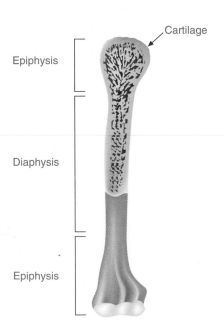

Fig. 3.37 Bone structure.

The outer surface of bone is covered with a layer of dense fibrous connective tissue called the *periosteum* into which are inserted muscles, tendons and ligaments for attachment. The inner surface of bone is covered by a delicate connective tissue layer, called the *endosteum*. Both these layers contain cells, which assist in the remodelling and repair of bone if it becomes damaged.

The function of bone and the skeletal system is to:

- Support the body
- Provide levers for movement
- Protect organs
- Maintain mineral levels in the body
- Produce blood cells (both red and white)

Joints

These are the articular surfaces of the ends of bones, always protected by a layer of cartilage (hyaline). The study of joints is termed *arthrology*. When joints become inflamed, this is termed *arthritis*.

Joints are places where different bones come into anatomical contact with each other:

- *Synarthroses* – are joints which are immovable, e.g. joints of the skull.
- *Diarthroses* – are joints where movement of adjacent bones can occur, and these are usually related to the limbs, e.g. synovial joints.
- *Amphiarthroses* – are joints which share some of the characteristics of the synarthroses and diarthroses but have limited movement, e.g. between the vertebrae of the spine.

Joints are further commonly classified as:

- *Fibrous* – no movement at all, also called suture joints, such as the bones of the skull.
- *Cartilaginous* – some movement to these. Examples are found where there are right and left sides, e.g. the lower jaw (mandibles) and in the pelvis.
- *Synovial* (Fig. 3.38) – plenty of movement to these joints. They also have other features:

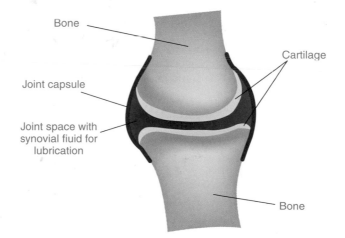

Bone

Cartilage

Joint capsule

Joint space with synovial fluid for lubrication

Bone

Fig. 3.38   Simple synovial joint.

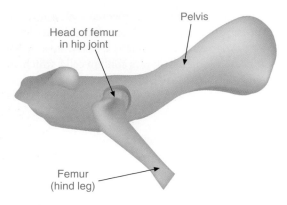

Fig. 3.39 Ball and socket joint.

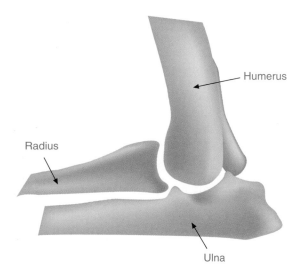

Fig. 3.40 Hinge joint.

    (a)   cartilage surfaces at bone ends
    (b)   joint membrane or capsule
    (c)   joint fluid for lubrication (synovial fluid).

Synovial joints may be called *simple* joints if they contain two articular surfaces, an example being the two bones which make up the shoulder joint. *Compound* joints have more than two articular surfaces, as in the elbow where three bones come together to form the joint.

The following simple and compound joints are generally recognized:

- Ball and socket (femur/acetabulum) (Fig. 3.39)
- Hinge (humerus/radius and ulna) (Fig. 3.40)
- Pivot (radius/ulna or atlas/axis) (Fig. 3.41)

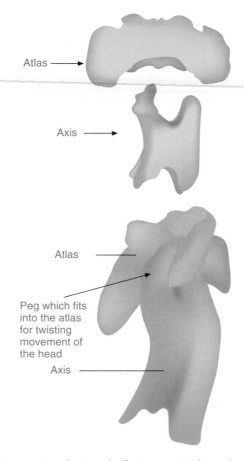

Atlas ⟶

Axis ⟶

Atlas ⟶

Peg which fits
into the atlas
for twisting
movement of
the head

Axis ⟶

Fig. 3.41   Pivot or rotatory joint showing the first two cervical vertebrae.

- Saddle (between phalanges of toes) (Fig. 3.42)
- Plane or gliding (between carpals/tarsals) (Fig. 3.42)
- Condylar (stifle or knee)

The stability of all synovial joints is improved by:

- Ligaments
- Surrounding muscles and tendons
- Well-shaped/fitting articular bone surfaces

The reproductive system

Reproduction refers to the formation of more individuals, from one parent (asexually) or from two parents (sexually).

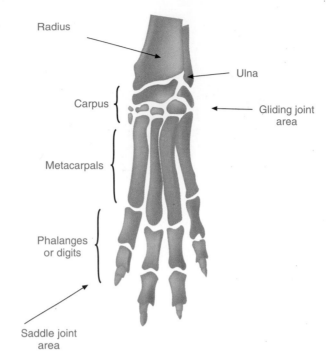

Fig. 3.42   Saddle and gliding joints – foot (foreleg).

Different species have evolved different processes, but in all species, from plants to mammals, reproduction is closely associated with protection against adverse conditions and survival over unfavourable periods.

Mammal reproduction is by a sexual process, and the male and female reproductive anatomy is very similar (Figs. 3.43 and 3.44).

The reproductive process

Every cell in every organism contains a set of instructions (genetic material) in chemical form for building the whole of the new organism. The set of instructions are called *chromosomes* and are situated in the nucleus of each cell. Reproduction is via special cells, produced only by the reproductive organs. Mammals have the most advanced reproductive systems in the animal kingdom. Not only do they have internal fertilisation they have internal development as well.

Internal development has the advantage that the female mammal does not have to remain in one place, as birds do when incubating their eggs, but can lead a reasonably normal life during pregnancy. This also assists in the survival of a species.

The female reproductive system has the following major functions:

- Production of the ova or egg.
- Receiving the male gametes or sperm.

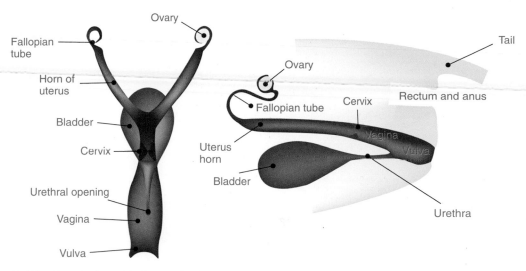

Fig. 3.43   Female dog and cat reproductive anatomy.

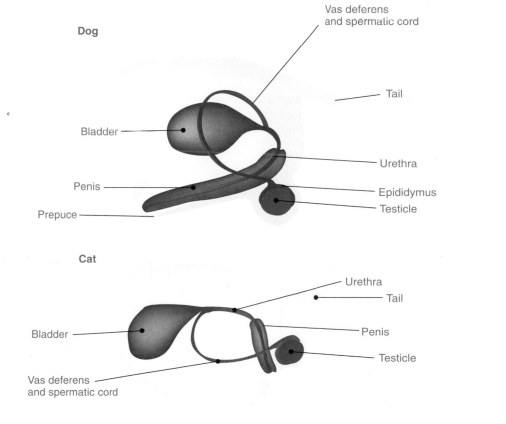

Fig. 3.44   Male dog and cat reproductive anatomy.

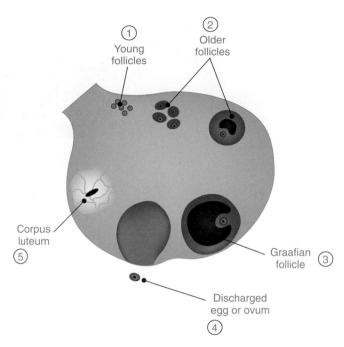

Fig. 3.45 Ovary and follicle. The stages of follicle development.

- Providing a suitable environment for the fertilisation of the egg by the sperm.
- Providing a safe place for the developing individuals/embryo.
- Providing food and nutrients to the developing individuals/embryo.

Production of ova (eggs)

The function of the ovary is to produce 'functional' eggs or *ova* and to act as an endocrine organ, producing hormones to maintain reproductive functions in the female.

Cells in the ovary group together to form *follicles* and follicular fluid (Fig. 3.45). Some of the follicles produce eggs. Their formation is similar to that of sperms in that meiosis occurs and each ovum will have only half the required number of chromosomes.

When the outer surface of the follicle ruptures, the follicular fluid and the mature ova are expelled. This is *ovulation*, and in some species, several ova are released at the same time. Eggs are passed into the *oviducts* or fallopian tubes which act as passageways to the uterus where, once fertilised by a sperm, the egg will implant and pregnancy (development of the embryo) takes place until the end of the gestation period and parturition (birth).

Production of sperm

The anatomy of the testes is shown in Fig. 3.46. In the testes, the walls of the seminiferous tubules consist of two types of cell:

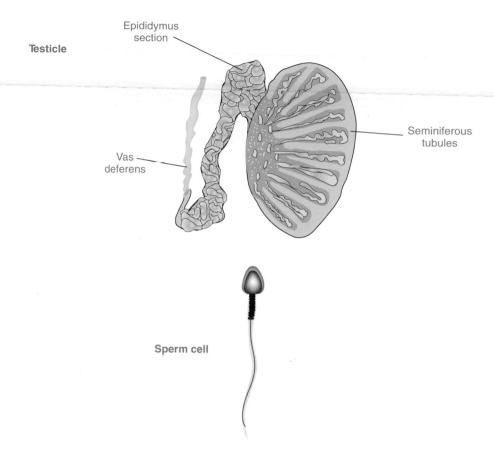

Fig. 3.46 Testicle and sperm cell.

(1) Those which produce sperm (*spermatogenic cells*) (Fig. 3.46).
(2) Those which produce fluid in which sperm may be supported and supplied with nutrients (*Sertoli cells*).

The testicles also produce the hormone *testosterone*.

The spermatogenic cells divide and from these *spermatids* are formed. These in turn become sperms by undergoing a series of changes including the formation of a tail section for movement. At this stage, they detach from the sperm-producing wall in the tubule and move into the epididymal duct for storage and to allow the sperm to mature. This leads to a sperm duct or *vas deferens*, which directs the sperm into the urethra.

The urethra leads to the penis, which is made up of erectile tissue, supported and encased in a heavy fibrous capsule. The penis contains the end section of the urethra which carries both urine and secretions containing sperm. It is the organ via which sperm is placed into the female reproductive tract.

Table 3.5 Species breeding data.

Species	Puberty	Oestrus	Gestation
Dog	7–12 months	Twice yearly	63–67 days
Cat	6–10 months	Every 21 days	63–65 days
Rabbit	3 months	Induced ovulation	30–33 days
Guinea pig	4–5 weeks	15–16-day cycle	60–72 days
Mouse	3–4 weeks	Every 4–5 days	19–21 days
Hamster	6–10 weeks	Every 4 days	15–22 days
Rat	6 weeks	Every 4–5 days	20–22 days

The breeding cycle

A female is said to be 'on heat' or 'in season', when she becomes attractive to the male, due to the secretion of pheromones (scent attractive to the male). Different species of animal will be in season at different times, so note must be taken of:

- The season – cats have a breeding season from January to September; rabbits breed from January to November
- Age
- Species variation

Table 3.5 provides breeding information for a range of species.

Oestrus

This is the period of sexual receptivity and, depending on species, may last from one to several days. During the rest of the oestrous cycle, the female does not accept the male's advances or allow mating. The cycle is made up of four or five stages, depending on the species and whether the animal is *polyoestrous* (cycles repeatedly like the cat, rat or hamster) or is *monoestrous* (cycles only once during the breeding season, like the dog).

The stages of oestrus

- *Anoestrus* – the end of the breeding season, with no activity on the part of the reproductive organs.
- *Pro-oestrus* – just before oestrus, FSH secretion causes the follicles to develop in the ovary. FSH stimulates the ovary to release increased amounts of oestrogen, causing changes to the reproductive tract and preparing for pregnancy.
- *Oestrus* – will accept a male. The release of the ova (ovulation) occurs. FSH levels decrease and LH increases, causing the ripened Graafian follicles to rupture, releasing the ova.
- *Metoestrus* – the period in which hormone activity fades and tissues are less active. If the ovum has been fertilised, the corpus luteum forms and produces progesterone,

which is responsible for maintaining pregnancy. Oestrogen secretions decrease. If pregnancy does not occur, the corpus luteum decreases in size, reducing the production of progesterone. This is followed by anoestrus and the cycle starts once more.

Signs of heat/oestrus

- Calling, can be very vocal, especially in cats
- More affectionate
- Restless
- Seeking the male animal
- Rolling and appearing submissive
- Swelling of the vaginal area
- Discharge from the vaginal area

Homeostasis

Homeostasis is the state of equilibrium in the body with respect to various functions and the chemical composition of fluids and tissues. The word 'homeostasis' means 'staying the same'. Some of the factors which must be kept the same are:

- Chemical constituents like glucose and electrolytes (salts)
- Osmotic pressure and the movement of fluid (water) and substances carried by this water
- Levels of the waste gas carbon dioxide
- Body temperature

Other products must be eliminated from the body because of their harmful effect. The most important of these are the nitrogenous waste products arising from protein metabolism and toxic substances released by micro-organisms that live in the body.

Internal environment

This refers to the immediate surroundings of the cells. The cells are surrounded by tiny channels and spaces filled with fluid, and the fluid can be identified by the following names:

- Intercellular (between)
- Extracellular interstitial
- Tissue fluid

The cells are provided with a medium in which they live, and this represents the organism's internal environment, which must be kept constant if the cells are to continue their vital functions. This fluid will return to the bloodstream eventually, either by osmotic pressure or via the lymph.

Other examples of homeostatic mechanisms in the body include the following:

- The regulation of sugar levels in the bloodstream. Sugar may be broken down and used as energy at the cellular level, stored in the liver as glycogen, converted to fat for storage or released into the bloodstream to top up the circulating levels.
- The aforementioned cannot be achieved without the various hormone chemical messengers provided by the organs of the endocrine system.
- The nervous system receives information from the body about all products and whether they are at the correct levels. If not, it sends a message to the organs concerned to rectify the situation.
- In order to control homeostasis, the body has feedback mechanisms. The sense organs feed back information to the brain, and from here, messages are sent to the relevant system or tissue for a response. The results of this response are then fed back to the brain, which decides on any subsequent action.

There is an important difference between homeostatic feedback and a voluntary or conscious control action by the body. In homeostasis, feedback is largely an unconscious activity – the animal is unaware that it is taking place.

Homeostasis is most highly developed in mammals and birds, probably as a result of their evolution. They are able to maintain a constant body temperature despite environmental temperature change. This is greatly assisted by feathers and fur for insulation.

Chapter 4
Basic Genetics

Summary

In this chapter, the learning outcomes are:

- To define the terms relating to basic genetics
- To identify the structure and function of chromosomes, genes and DNA
- To identify and describe the stages of cell division – mitosis and meiosis

What is genetics?

Genetics is the study of heredity – how characteristics are passed from parent to off-spring and subsequently down the generations.

Why is genetics important?

Studying genetics allows us to identify dominant characteristics; it allows us to identify genes that cause particular diseases, and it allows us to map the genetic code (genome) for certain species, e.g. dogs and humans.

Important events in the history of genetics

Gregor Mendel (1822–1884) is said to be the father of modern genetics. Mendel was an Austrian monk that lived in the nineteenth century. He conducted many investigations on pea plants and made detailed notes about their inherited characteristics which were published at the time through the Brünn Society for the Study of Natural History. At the time, his investigations were disregarded but became of more importance 40 years subsequently by which time Mendel had died. Mendel's theories were brought forwards by the Dutch scientist Hugo De Vries (1848–1935).

Animal Biology and Care, Third Edition. Sue Dallas and Emily Jewell.
© 2014 John Wiley & Sons, Ltd. Published 2014 by John Wiley & Sons, Ltd.
Companion Website: www.wiley.com/go/dallas/animal-biology-care

Mendel's investigations with pea plants culminated in him establishing two laws relating to inheritance and forming the basis of today's modern genetics. Mendelian genetics were the cornerstone to today's advances in genetics.

Mendel's first law

Mendel's first law is also referred to as the 'Law of Segregation'. This law states that every individual has a pair of alleles for any particular trait and that each parent passes a randomly selected copy of one allele to its offspring. The trait exhibited in the offspring will depend on which of the alleles received from the parents are dominant, e.g. colour of an animal's fur.

Mendel's second law

Mendel's second law is also called the 'Law of Inheritance'. It states that separate genes of separate traits are passed independently of each other from parent to offspring. Mendel stated that different traits shown in a species are inherited independently of each other. This is now known only to be true when genes are not linked to each other.

Chromosomes, genes and DNA

In an earlier chapter, it was said that the nucleus of the cell contains the chromosomes and that chromosomes are rod-shaped components containing DNA. DNA contains the genetic code to the characteristics an animal possesses. It is due to this genetic code that DNA can produce exact copies of itself and instructions can be passed on to new cells that form in the body. Chromosomes are always found in pairs in the nucleus.

The shape of the DNA molecule within the nucleus is one of its most significant features. It is known as the double helix and was discovered in 1953 by James Watson and Francis Crick and was one of the most notable discoveries of the twentieth century. The helix shape is brought about by two strands being linked across the middle to form 'stairs'. When stretched out, the DNA of a cell can stretch to 1.5 m in length.

Each linkage strand within the double helix structure is simply a long line of chemical units called *nucleotides*. A nucleotide consists of a sugar molecule and a phosphate molecule linked to a DNA base. There are four different types of DNA bases which are represented by the letters A, G, C and T. Each single strand of DNA can contain any sequence of these letters. On the opposite strand of DNA will be a similar sequence of the letters, and if one side of the strand is known, then the other side can be predicted as the nucleotides always exist in set pairs: A always pairs with T and C always pairs with G.

Therefore, if the code on one strand is:

AATCGCTAATGCCGGAT

then the code on the opposite strand is:

TTAGCGATTACGGCCTA

Table 4.1   Number of chromosomes in different species.

Species	Number of chromosomes
Human	46
Chimpanzee	48
Horse	64
Dog	76
Cat	38

The base pairs are attached to a *sugar phosphate backbone* which comprises the longitudinal strands on the helix. The base pairs are:

A = adenine   T = thymine
G = guanine   C = cytosine

As already mentioned, DNA is stored in the nucleus of a cell in structures called chromosomes. The number of chromosomes in each species of animal is different and specific to that species – Table 4.1.

The DNA on the chromosomes is split into specific segments called genes. Genes are the single unit of heredity. Many characteristics can be determined by a single gene. Genes control all aspects of the body, whether it is the coat, hair or eye colour; rate of bone growth; or the ability of the blood to clot. Unfortunately, genes are responsible for many diseases and disorders as well, which are called inherited factors.

Each gene has its own allocated place on a particular chromosome, called the gene locus. Genes exist in pairs, just like chromosomes. Therefore, each chromosome carries two copies of a gene. The copies may not be the same, and in this case, genes that occupy the same gene locus on a chromosome are called alleles.

Genetic terms

Table 4.2 can be used as a glossary of commonly used genetic terms.

Cell division

There are two methods of cell division, depending on the cells involved.

Mitosis

Mitosis is the type of cell division that results in the production of two identical daughter cells, each containing an identical set of chromosomes compared to the parent cell.

Table 4.2 Genetics glossary of terms.

Term	Definition
Genetics	The science of heredity, i.e. how characteristics are passed on from parents to offspring
Meiosis	Cell division process to form daughter cells containing half the original number of chromosomes – exclusive to sex cells
Mitosis	Cell division process to form new cells containing the same number of chromosomes as the parent cell
DNA	Deoxyribonucleic acid
RNA	Ribonucleic acid
Chromosomes	Structures within the nucleus of a cell that contain all the information for the characteristics of an individual
Genes	The basic unit of inheritance for any characteristic – lengths of DNA that contain specific codes for particular proteins
Locus	The particular location of a gene on a chromosome
Allele	Different versions of the same gene occupying the same locus on the chromosome, e.g. coat colour
Genotype	The genetic make-up of an animal
Phenotype	The physical expression of genotype – i.e. the appearance of the animal, e.g. coat colour
Dominant	Genes that are expressed in the phenotype even when only one allele is present. Dominant alleles suppress other alleles and are represented by capital letters, e.g. B in the genotypes BB and Bb
Recessive	These alleles are only expressed in the phenotype when both alleles are present and are represented by lower-case letters, e.g. b in Bb and bb. The recessive characteristic will only be shown in the case of bb
Co-dominant	Both alleles of a gene are expressed
Homozygous	Both alleles of a particular gene are the same, e.g. BB or bb
Heterozygous	Alleles of a particular gene are different, e.g. Bb
Masked genes/epistasis	Some genes have an overwhelming effect on other genes and can block the expression of alleles on a different locus, e.g. albino gene blocks coat colour gene
Mimic genes	This occurs when two or more distinctly different genes produce similar bodily effects. Mimic genes are often expressed in species that want to look like more toxic versions of themselves
Rogue genes	Produce bad or life-threatening effects on the animal, e.g. extra toes, deafness in white gene animals, eyesight defects like the Siamese gene
Lethal factors	Genes that are not compatible with life and so the animal dies if one of these genes is present

Mitosis occurs in all body cells (somatic cells) except the sex cells (gametes). The original number of chromosomes is known as the diploid number.

Before a cell divides, copies of each chromosome form alongside the originals and then separate from the originals. As a cell divides, a full set of chromosomes collect at each end to form part of the two new cell nuclei (Fig. 4.1).

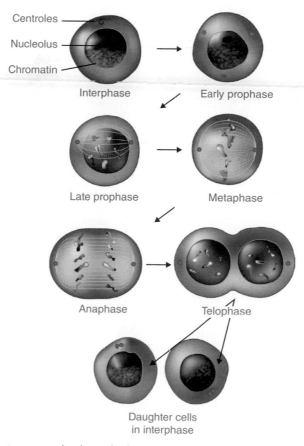

Centroles

Nucleolus

Chromatin

Interphase   Early prophase

Late prophase   Metaphase

Anaphase   Telophase

Daughter cells
in interphase

Fig. 4.1 Mitosis. Source: Dorland's Medical Dictionary for Health Consumers (2007). Reproduced with permission of Elsevier.

Meiosis

Meiosis is the type of cell division that results in the production of gamete cells. Meiosis only occurs in the ovaries or testes. Each daughter cell produced contains only half the number of chromosomes when compared to the parent cell. This half number of chromosomes is known as the haploid number. The result of meiosis is that each sperm and each egg contains one member of each pair of chromosomes. The union of a sperm with an egg at fertilization produces a fertilized egg with the usual diploid number of chromosomes (Fig 4.2).

The phases of mitosis and meiosis can be remembered using the acronym IPMAT:

- I   Interphase
- P   Prophase
- M   Metaphase
- A   Anaphase
- T   Telophase

The final division in both processes is known as cytokinesis.

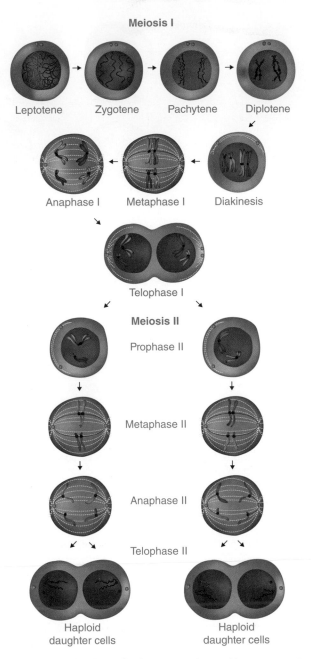

Meiosis I

Leptotene   Zygotene   Pachytene   Diplotene

Anaphase I   Metaphase I   Diakinesis

Telophase I

Meiosis II

Prophase II

Metaphase II

Anaphase II

Telophase II

Haploid
daughter cells

Haploid
daughter cells

Fig. 4.2   Meiosis. Source: Dorland's Medical Dictionary for Health Consumers (2007). Reproduced with permission of Elsevier.

Comparison of mitosis and meiosis

Table 4.3 Comparison of mitosis and meiosis.

Mitosis	Meiosis
Division of a body cell to form new body cells	Division of cells in the sex organs (testes or ovaries) to form sex cells (gametes)
The daughter cell carries identical gene information to the parent cell	The daughter cells give each new cell half the number of genes present
Both cells are referred to as diploid	Both cells are referred to as haploid
	Takes place only in the testes and ovaries

Breeding and genetics

Genetic studies have become more and more important in relation to the breeding of pedigree animals. There is considerable focus in these times on inherited diseases that are completely avoidable if disease-free animals are bred from. Responsible breeders will test for these diseases and avoid breeding from affected stock.

Anyone that is considering breeding from an animal should research the animals and make careful choices in the selection of a mate in order to avoid producing offspring that are carrying inherited disease(s).

It is important to be aware of the following terms when discussing breeding:

- *Pedigree* – mother and father of the same breed with written pedigree from the owner tracing ancestors (pedigree chart).
- *Crossbred* – mother and father were of different breeds. They may both be purebred, making the offspring a 'first cross'. This means the size and behaviour of the offspring are reasonably predictable still. This type of breeding is becoming more popular to create fashionable/designer breeds, e.g. Labrador × Poodle – Labradoodle and Pug × Beagle – Puggle.
- *Mongrel* – if the same female is mated with an already crossbred male, the offspring would be mongrels. This means the size and behaviour of the offspring are unpredictable.
- *Inbreeding* – mating for specific characteristics. It involves mating individuals more closely related than animals chosen from other bloodlines, for example, father/daughter and brother/sister.
- *Line breeding* – is a form of inbreeding but animals are not so closely related. It is mating within certain family lines and maintains a relationship with a particular ancestor for particular characteristics.
- *Outbreeding* – breeding individuals less closely related chosen at random from available animals.

Table 4.4 identifies a glossary of terms relating to breeding.

Table 4.4   Glossary of breeding-related terms.

Term	Definition
Sire	The father
Dam	The mother
Seasonally monoestrous	An animal that has one reproductive cycle in a breeding season
Seasonally polyoestrous	An animal that has more than one reproductive cycle within a breeding season
Pro-oestrus	The first part of a reproductive cycle where a female starts to become attractive to males but does not mate
Oestrus	The second part of the reproductive cycle characterized by sexual activity in animals and ovulation
Metoestrus	Period after ovulation where corpora lutea are formed and produce progesterone for maintaining pregnancy
Interoestrus	The short period of time between each reproductive cycle in one breeding season
Anoestrus	A long period of reproductive inactivity between reproductive cycles in between breeding seasons
Season	The time at which an animal is ready to mate, i.e. oestrus
Puberty	The time at which an animal is sexually mature and able to breed
Adolescence	The growth phase prior to puberty usually equating to teenage years
Misalliance	A mating that has occurred that is unplanned/unwanted
Gestation	Pregnancy
Pseudopregnancy	False pregnancy
Parturition	Labour and birth
Dystocia	Difficulty/problems giving birth
Lactation	The period of milk production in mammals
Neonate	Newborn animal
Colostrum	The first milk produced by the mother which contains antibodies
Weaning	The process of transferring young onto solid foods from milk

Chapter 5
Body Areas

Summary

In this chapter, the learning outcomes are:

- To be able to name the different body cavities
- To be able to identify the boundaries of the different body cavities
- To be able to identify the main organs of the different body cavities

When describing the location of a part of the body, it is helpful to be able to identify more accurately the part of the body using veterinary terminology. A number of areas are described in order to aid these descriptions.

Thoracic cavity

The thoracic cavity is found within the chest. Its boundaries are as follows:

- *Cranial or anterior* – the thoracic inlet through which the trachea and oesophagus pass
- *Dorsal* – the thoracic vertebrae and joining muscles
- *Ventral* – the sternum
- *Lateral* – the ribs and intercostal muscles
- *Caudal or posterior* – the diaphragm

The heart and lungs are located within the thoracic cavity. The heart is surrounded by the *pericardium* which is a double membrane layer designed to protect the heart.

Abdominal cavity

The abdominal cavity is found between the thoracic cavity and pelvic region of the animal. Its cranial boundary is the diaphragm and its caudal limit is the pelvic opening. Dorsally are the lumbar vertebrae and the diaphragm. Lateral and ventral boundaries

Animal Biology and Care, Third Edition. Sue Dallas and Emily Jewell.
© 2014 John Wiley & Sons, Ltd. Published 2014 by John Wiley & Sons, Ltd.
Companion Website: www.wiley.com/go/dallas/animal-biology-care

are the abdominal muscles. The abdominal cavity contains the stomach, liver, gall bladder, intestines, pancreas and kidneys.

Pelvic region

There is no physical barrier that splits the abdominal cavity and the pelvis, hence why this area is often referred to as the pelvic region. Its cranial opening is the pelvic inlet and the caudal opening is the pelvic outlet. Dorsally are the bones of the pelvis (pubis and ischium), and the lateral boundaries are muscles or ligaments. The pelvic region protects the bladder, the sex organs and the rectum.

Cavity linings

Body cavities are lined with a *serous membrane*. This is a smooth, shiny membrane which produces a watery fluid to lubricate between two tissue surfaces and prevent friction:

- In the thoracic cavity, the lining is the *pleura*. If the pleura becomes inflamed, then the animal is suffering from pleurisy.
- In the abdominal and pelvic cavities, the lining is the *peritoneum*. If the peritoneum becomes inflamed, then the animal is suffering from peritonitis which can be extremely serious.

More veterinary terminology can be found in the Appendix at the back of the book.

Section 2
Animal Health and Husbandry

Chapter 6
Animal Welfare

Summary

In this chapter, the learning outcomes are:

- To be able to define the term animal welfare
- To describe how to assess animal welfare through identification of the good and poor indicators of animal welfare
- To identify the main pieces of Animal Welfare Legislation, notably the Animal Welfare Act 2006 and the Five Animal Needs alongside a number of other pieces of legislation
- To describe the main rules of the Pet Travel Scheme
- To investigate types of animal welfare organisation and develop understanding of these organisations through further research on the internet
- To briefly examine the concept of animal rights

Animal welfare is a term that is frequently used within the animal industry and regard for an animal's welfare has to be paramount for anyone caring for or working with animals. There are many important strands to animal welfare, and it is important to know what the term means and how the welfare of an animal can be promoted.

Definition of animal welfare

> Animal welfare is the physical and psychological state of an animal as regards its attempt to cope with its environment.
>
> Professor Donald M Broom (1991), Colleen Macleod
> Professor of Animal Welfare, University of Cambridge, UK

It logically follows therefore that the factors that affect an animal's welfare are not only the environment in which it lives but also the treatment it receives from its owners/carers/keepers and the quality of the animal's life.

Animal Biology and Care, Third Edition. Sue Dallas and Emily Jewell.
© 2014 John Wiley & Sons, Ltd. Published 2014 by John Wiley & Sons, Ltd.
Companion Website: www.wiley.com/go/dallas/animal-biology-care

Consider the following cases which could occur:

Case 1

A 6-year-old brood bitch is kept in the house of her owner, is provided with a nice warm bed, is given the best diet for her breed, has access to fresh water at all times, is sufficiently exercised every day and is played with to stimulate her mind, and the owner has bred from her every year for the past 3 years and plans to continue to do so. Consider whether the bitch's welfare needs are being met in terms of quality of life.

Case 2

A small rescue centre has been given a pair of female ferrets at a weekend when there is minimal staffing and several volunteers. One of the volunteers has been told to find some housing until the manager is in work on Monday. The volunteer places the ferrets in an empty hutch and run that is large enough for the ferrets. The hutch that the ferrets are in is opposite a bank of hutches that currently houses rabbits. Consider how the welfare of (a) the rabbits and (b) the ferrets is affected by the actions of the volunteer.

Case 3

A young couple own 1 Siamese cat. The cat was the centre of their world until recently a baby was born. The cat is fed each day and has access to water, but the food bowl is often overflowing and the water is not always replaced each day. The cat has access to a litter tray and also outside if necessary, but the litter tray is not always cleaned on a daily basis. The cat used to sleep on the owner's bed prior to the arrival of the baby and is now only allowed in a certain area of the house. Consider how the cat's welfare has been affected by the arrival of the baby.

How is animal welfare assessed?

To assess the welfare of an animal, it is important to consider the whole animal and consider the good and bad aspects of welfare.

Indicators of good welfare

- A variety of normal behaviours shown
- Physiological indicators of pleasure
- Behavioural indicators of pleasure

This can be difficult to assess as an animal's behaviour can sometimes mask how it is really feeling. Most assessments of animal welfare tend to focus on the poor indicators of animal welfare.

Indicators of poor welfare

There are two types of indicators related to poor welfare:

(1) Indicators relating to a failure to cope:
  - (a) Reduced life expectancy
  - (b) Reduced ability to grow or breed
  - (c) Increased disease
  - (d) Reduced survival of offspring
  - (e) Reduction in production output (e.g. milk, eggs)
(2) Extreme efforts involved in coping or attempting to cope:
  - (a) Extreme changes in physiology – the stress response is put into action.
  - (b) Changes in behaviour – abnormal behaviours displayed and reluctance to perform normal behaviours.

It is important to remember that an animal's welfare affects both the physical and psychological status of the animal.

Animal welfare legislation

The law acts as a framework of guidelines for people to work within to uphold professional standards in relation to society. It is the responsibility of all people who work with animals to maintain a practical and working knowledge of the law relating to the animals and the industry which they are working in as well as always working within that law. The legislation in the UK refers to both Acts of Parliament and Regulations.

Laws (also known as statutes) – are created by the Parliament. Presented as draft legislation in the form of a bill, they are debated initially in the House of Commons and the House of Lords. They are each then considered by a specifically formed parliamentary committee, before finally receiving the queen's signature to become law and being placed on the Statute Book as an Act of Parliament.

Regulations (orders) – these detail the technical implications of laws. The relevant government minister adds regulations to the legislation. This information is a supplement to existing law and must have the approval of the Parliament.

Welfare codes – must also have parliamentary approval. Failure to comply with the provisions of a code is not in itself an offence, but could be used in evidence if prosecuted.

In addition to the discussions made earlier, we must abide by the standards set by the European Union (EU) which have been incorporated into, and take precedence over, the UK law.

The purpose of any animal-related legislation is:

- To ensure the health, welfare and protection of the animals through setting minimum husbandry requirements
- To protect the public
- To set standards and provide a framework of guidelines for the control of licensing in certain areas of the animal industry

Animal Welfare Act 2006

The Animal Welfare Act (AWA) 2006 is without doubt the most significant piece of legislation concerning animal welfare to be published in recent times. It takes several outdated pieces of legislation such as the Protection of Animals Act 1911 and the Abandonment of Animals Act 1960 and brings them together with additional information to produce a piece of legislation more relevant to today's society. There are still certain aspects that are to be reviewed, and the act will be added to subsequently as eventually all existing animal laws will be replaced and regulated for under the AWA.

The AWA applies to all vertebrate animals with the exclusion of humans. One of the most important aims of the act is that it relates specifically to pet owners to ensure that they have a legal duty of care to meet the five animal welfare needs of their pet(s). The AWA is also applicable to all people who work with animals and keep animals for breeding or working purposes whether in a zoo, aquarium, circus, farm park, rescue centre, kennels or veterinary practice.

The Five Animal Needs were previously known as the Five Freedoms of Animal Welfare. The Five Freedoms were created in 1963 in relation to farm livestock, and over the years, they have been applied to all animals kept in captivity and have now been amended to be known as the Five Animal Needs. By meeting the needs, it is ensured that people are caring for those animals properly and are promoting responsible pet ownership.

The Five Animal Needs

- An animal should have somewhere suitable to live.
- An animal should have a proper diet, including fresh water.
- An animal should have the ability to express normal behaviour.
- An animal should have its needs to be housed with, or apart from, other animals met.
- An animal should have protection from, and treatment of, illness and injury.

When establishing how the needs for an animal can be met, an owner should think about what the animal would have in its natural environment in terms of housing, feeding and how it relates to other animals. By meeting these basic needs, the animal should be able to display the normal behavioural repertoire for that species. Due to the fact that animals are kept in captivity, whether as pets, working animals, production animals or visitor attractions, owners/keepers of those animals have a responsibility to ensure that the animal(s) remains healthy and protected against illness and disease, and this includes preventative treatments as well as reactive treatments.

The five welfare needs are important to animal welfare as they provide a framework on which to provide advice and guidance to owners/carers/keepers.

The five welfare needs also provide a framework for organisations such as the RSPCA to step in prior to animal suffering occurring which was not possible under the previous legislation. Environmental Health Officers also now have the power to issue improvement notices and prosecute if an animal is being mistreated. The AWA allows improvement notices to be issued prior to seizure of any animals, and so, owners/carers/keepers have a chance to resolve any situation in the first instance.

The key areas addressed by the AWA are that animals may not be sold or given as prizes to children aged under 16 and that separate sections have been incorporated to address the contentious and emotive issues of tail docking, animal fighting, mutilation and animal poisoning.

A person or persons that are successfully prosecuted under the AWA may be disqualified from owning/keeping/dealing in/transporting a specific type of animal (e.g. dogs) or be disqualified from owning/keeping/dealing in/transporting all animals, depending upon the nature of the offence. They can also face up to a year in prison and/or a £20 000 fine.

Animal-related legislation that has still yet to be reviewed includes:

Breeding of Dogs Acts 1973 and 1991 as amended by the Breeding and Sale of Dogs (Welfare) Act 1999

- The breeding and selling of dogs require a local authority licence under the 1973 Act, amended by the 1999 Act. In order to gain a licence, animals must be suitably accommodated, fed, exercised and protected from disease and fire. Local authorities have extensive powers to check on the standards of health, accommodation and welfare (checking the five needs are met) of these animals, and local authorities are empowered to enter and inspect the premises whether licensed or unlicensed.
- The term 'breeding establishment' refers to any premises where more than two bitches are kept for the purpose of breeding animals for selling. The 1999 Act ensures that 'puppy farms' are regulated by the use of recorded information on sales and identification. The 1999 Act also caters for 'one-off' breeders and states that those breeders that do not produce any more than five litters in a 12-month period do not require a licence.
- The legislation places limits on when a bitch can be bred from and how many litters she can have in order to protect her welfare. Bitches should not be bred from until they are 1 year of age in order to allow sufficient growth and development of themselves. They cannot have more than one litter in a 12-month period and also should not have more than six litters over their lifetime. This aims to prevent bitches from becoming brood factories. In order to follow these legislative requirements, the breeder is required to keep breeding records. The puppies produced by a breeder can only be sold at the breeding premises or at a licensed pet shop.

Riding Establishments Acts 1964 and 1970

- Riding establishments must be licensed by the local authority who can impose certain conditions on the premises. When inspecting a riding establishment, the local authority will take into account the suitability and experience of the applicant, the accommodation and the grazing provision for the horses and also check that the five needs are met for the horses. They will also check the suitability of the horses kept at the premises and ensure there is a provision for evacuation to occur in case of a fire.

Animal Boarding Establishments Act 1963

- In any establishment (including private dwellings) where animals (specifically cats and dogs) are boarded as a business, the local authority has a requirement to inspect and license those premises as being suitable and meet the animal's welfare needs under this legislation.
- The following conditions apply under this legislation:
  - Records must be kept of animal arrivals and departures and details of owners
  - Suitable accommodation must be provided
  - Adequate and appropriate supplies of food and water must be available
  - Exercise facilities must be provided
  - Animals must be protected from disease and risk of fire
- In order to ensure the conditions of the licence are met, the local authority can enter the premises at any time. Licences are renewed annually.

Dangerous Wild Animals Act 1976, amended 2010

- The Dangerous Wild Animals Act (DWAA) 1976 aims to ensure that private individuals who keep dangerous wild animals do so safely in a way that creates no risk to the public. The act was introduced due to the sudden desire of the public to begin keeping more exotic animals, and there was a concern for the welfare of the animals and also the safety of the public. Individuals must be licensed to keep animals that appear on the Schedule to the act which is available on the Department for Environment, Food and Rural Affairs (DEFRA) website. The government may amend the list at any time, and it is the responsibilities of animal owners/keepers to keep themselves familiarised with the Schedule.
- Inspections are carried out by authorised veterinary surgeons who then report to the local authority as to whether a licence should or should not be issued.
- Any person that holds a licence must:
  - Be 18+ years of age
  - Hold sufficient liability insurance
  - Meet the welfare needs of the animal
- The DWAA was amended in March 2010 and the main changes were:
  - A licence being valid for a maximum of 2 years instead of 1 year
  - New licences coming into force immediately upon being granted
- Animals kept under the DWAA are also subject to protection under the AWA 2006.

Dangerous Dogs Act 1991, amended 1997

- After an increase in the number of attacks on people by dogs in the 1980s and 1990s, some fatal, the government introduced laws, making it more difficult to own and import into the UK the following breeds of dog:
  - American Pit Bull Terrier
  - Japanese Tosa
  - Dogo Argentino
  - Fila Brasileiro
- The act lists specific rules that owners of the named breeds of dangerous dog must abide by:
  - Notify the police of ownership
  - Obtain a certificate of exemption from the police, which is only issued once the dog has been neutered and permanently identified with either a microchip or another method such as a tattoo
  - The dog must be covered by third-party liability insurance
  - In public places, the dog must always be on a lead and muzzled
  - The dog must not be solely taken out by anyone under 16 years of age
  - The dog should not be sold, exchanged or abandoned; otherwise, prosecution can occur
  - It is an offence to breed from these dogs
- It is important to note that **any** dog dangerously out of control and a risk to the general public comes under the remit of this act. The person in charge of a dog that has inflicted injury could be prosecuted and face an unlimited fine or prison sentence.
- During 2012, consultation began on reviewing this act to ensure it is fit for purpose in today's society.

Zoo Licensing Act 1981, amended 2002

- The Zoo Licensing Act 1981 sets out how zoos in Great Britain are inspected and licensed in order to ensure that zoos are safe for the public to visit, that high standards of animal welfare are implemented and that zoos make a contribution to conservation of wildlife. European Council Directive 1999/22/EC is also implemented in the UK through this piece of legislation.
- Under this act, the term zoo refers to a collection of wild animals that are on display to the public for educational purposes. If this collection opens to the public for 7 or more days in any 1 year, then they must apply for a zoo licence.
- Local authorities are responsible for issuing licences to zoological collections, following an inspection of the premises with an authorized Secretary of State Zoo Inspector. Licences are renewed on a four yearly basis with interim checks during the period that the licence is held.
- Any vertebrate animals kept in zoos are also subject to protection under the AWA 2006.

The Performing Animals (Regulation) Act 1925

- The AWA 2006 covers the welfare of performing animals under its general provisions to avoid suffering.
- The training and exhibition of performing animals are regulated by the 1925 Act which requires trainers and exhibitors of such animals to be registered with the local authority. Under this act, the police and officers of local authorities, who may include a vet, are empowered to enter premises where animals are being trained and exhibited. If cruelty and neglect are detected, the training or exhibition of the animals can be prohibited and the trainer's registration suspended.
- The act was introduced to cover circus animals in the first instance but now extends to all public exhibitions of animals. Exceptions to the act are animals trained for sporting purposes, military or police dog work or display.

Pet Animals Act 1951, amended 1983

- The Pet Animals Act protects the welfare of those animals sold as pets through business premises. Any pet shop must be licensed by the local authority following an inspection by authorised personnel to ensure that welfare needs are met through the provision of:
  - Suitable accommodation with correct reference to heating, lighting, etc.
  - Adequate and appropriate supplies of food and water
  - Appropriate exercise facilities
  - Protection of the animals from disease
  - Functional emergency and fire precautions for the premises are in place
  - Suitable checks and observations throughout the day
- Animals may only be sold once they have been weaned and a suitable age for sale has been reached. This will vary according to the species being sold, but the seller should ensure that the animal is healthy and feeding properly.
- Conditions may be attached to the licence, and the local authority is empowered to enter the premises and inspect at any time. Licences may be suspended or withdrawn if the terms of the licence are not being adhered to.
- The act was amended in 1983, making it illegal to sell pets in public places.

Other examples of legislation relevant to animal care/management situations

There is much legislation in existence that relates to animals whether to protect them or the public. Some of the most relevant acts are summarised in the following section.

Animal Health Act 1981 amended 2002 including the Rabies (Importation of Dogs, Cats and Other Mammals) Order 1974

- The Animal Health Act 1981 covers a range of situations relating to animal health including biosecurity, cleaning and disinfection, identification of animals, movement of animal carcasses, animals entering the food chain, transport of live animals, identification of dogs in public places (must wear a collar with an identity tag stating name and address of owner), National Contingency Plan relating to specific diseases and import and export of animals.

- The Animal Health Act 1981 makes provision for dealing with notifiable diseases named in Section 88 of the act. Any person that is in possession of an animal that is suspected or confirmed as having a notifiable disease must report to the police.
- The Animal Health Act also allows the appropriate authorities to deal with suspect or confirmed rabies cases, under the Rabies (Control) Order 1974. It allows government officers to remove affected or suspected animals and those that have been exposed to the infection. The orders and regulations covered by the Rabies (Control) Order 1974 include:
  - o Reporting of suspected or actual cases of rabies to the DEFRA, the local authority and the police
  - o Declaring the place where the suspected animal is identified as an infected area. This can also result in control of movement on and off the premises and prevent any gathering of animals in the local area
  - o Destruction of an infected animal by authorized veterinary personnel.
- The Rabies (Importation of Dogs, Cats and Other Mammals) Order 1974 also provides the Secretary of State with the power to extend the quarantine period of any animal detained at quarantine premises if:
  - o An outbreak of rabies occurs at quarantine premises
  - o An animal in quarantine is suspected of being infected by rabies
- The Rabies (Control) Order 1974 also applies to suspected cases in quarantine premises. Movement of animals into and out of the premises would stop, including those animals covered by the requirements of the Pet Travel Scheme (PETS).
- The Animal Health Act 2002 amendment provides additional guidance on foot-and-mouth disease and other diseases as required and also provides additional powers for dealing with transmissible spongiform encephalopathies such as BSE and scrapie. Amendments have been made to powers of enforcement and also include further guidance on biosecurity as well as specific offences against animals.

The Pet Travel Scheme

The PETS is the arrangement that allows pet animals (dogs, cats and ferrets) from certain countries to enter the UK without going into quarantine, providing that they comply with the rules under the scheme. It also allows pet owners from the UK to take and return with their pets (dogs, cats and ferrets) having visited EU countries and some non-EU (listed) qualifying countries, providing they have also followed the criteria of the scheme as follows:

- The animal must be fitted with a microchip
- The animal must be vaccinated against rabies (providing they have met the minimum age for vaccination). Subsequent rabies boosters must be kept up to date.

The final vaccination must have been administered at least 21 days before the date of re-entry to the UK. The day of vaccination is counted as day 0. The 21-day wait for re-entry was introduced in January 2012

- The animal must have a blood test to ensure that the vaccine has given it a satisfactory level of protection against rabies
- The **owner** must organise and possess the relevant documentation:
  - for an EU country, an EU pet passport is required. A passport can also be issued in Croatia, Norway, San Marino, Switzerland and Gibraltar
  - for a non-EU country, it is necessary to obtain an official third-country veterinary certificate – different certificates apply for different situations, so it is important to check that the right one is issued
  - animals from unlisted countries must spend 6 months in quarantine on arrival in the UK
  - travel to the Isle of Man and the Channel Islands does not require a pet passport
  - pet passports can only be issued by official veterinary surgeons in the UK, and it is important to ensure that all relevant sections are completed correctly
- If you are re-entering from a non-EU country, the animal must have a blood test to ensure a satisfactory level of protection against rabies. The blood sample cannot be taken until day 30 after the final rabies vaccination was administered (remembering that the day of administration is day 0). Currently, there is a 3-month waiting period for an animal to enter the UK once the blood sample has been taken and indicated a satisfactory level of protection. The only exception to this is if an animal was vaccinated and blood tested in the EU and was issued with an EU pet passport before travelling to the unlisted country
- Before re-entry to the UK, dogs specifically must be treated against tapeworms – specifically *Echinococcus multilocularis* between 24 and 120 hours (1–5 days) before it is scheduled to enter the UK. The active ingredient against this tapeworm is Praziquantel, and the product used should be checked to ensure that it contains this ingredient. Dogs travelling from the following countries are exempt from this step – Norway, Finland, Ireland and Malta. There is no longer a mandatory need for animals to be treated for ticks prior to re-entry to the UK
- Arrangements must be made for the pet animal to travel with an approved transport company on an authorised route prior to entry to the UK
- If it is found at any stage that the PETS has not been complied with, then the animal must enter quarantine for a period of 6 months

The rules are to keep the UK free from rabies and certain other exotic diseases. Although the UK has been free of rabies for many years, certain parasitic diseases are on the increase, and it is vital that there is an effective system in place to monitor animals entering into the UK.

Up-to-date information relating to the PETS can be found on the DEFRA website, and this should always be checked thoroughly prior to travel as rules vary according to the intended country of travel or re-entry – for example, cats travelling from Australia must have a certificate showing protection against Hendra disease, and cats and dogs entering from the Malaysian Peninsula must have certificates showing protection against Nipah disease. The scheme also applies to assistance dogs such as guide dogs and hearing dogs. If five or more animals are being moved at any one time, then certain conditions apply, and these can be found on the DEFRA website.

It must be noted that if animals are permanently moving for sale or rehoming, then movement must be according to conditions of the Balai Directive 92/65/EEC. The Balai Directive applies to animals used for display, education, conservation or research including laboratory animals. Equid species are exempt from this directive as there is specific legislation in existence relating to the movement of such species. The details of the Balai Directive can be found on the DEFRA website.

Guard Dogs Act 1975

- The Guard Dogs Act exists to ensure that dogs used to protect property are used safely and are under control so as not to put the general public at risk.
- Notices must be displayed advising that guard dogs are on the premises, especially at the entrance to the premises.
- Guard dogs should only be off the lead if a person capable of controlling the dog is present. Guard dogs should not be left to freely roam the premises.
- Owners of guard dogs can be liable for any injuries to people under the Animals Act 1971 unless they are covered by an exemption under this act.

Animals Act 1971

- This act covers civil liability for damage that has been caused by animals, including damage, death and injury caused to people, property and livestock.
- The owner of a dangerous animal must take precautions to ensure that there is no opportunity for the animal to inflict damage as stated by this law. If a dog kills or harms farm animals, farmers are entitled to protect the stock in their care. For example, if a dog is found harming sheep, the farmer may kill the dog but must report the incident to the police.
- If the owner of the animal is under 16, then the parent of the owner becomes liable. The owner is classed as the person in possession of the animal at the time of the injurious incident. There are exemptions from this in certain circumstances such as if the person suffering the injury was proven to be at fault or if the livestock harmed had strayed on to land where the dog was authorised to be present by the owner of the land.
- The term livestock under this act also includes captive game birds as well as farm livestock.

Dog Control Orders Regulations 2006

- These orders replace the Dog (Fouling of Land) Act 1996.
- In 2006, Dog Control Orders were introduced and can be put in place on an area of land in order to control:

- o Dog fouling
- o Restricting access of dogs to certain areas of land (e.g. beaches)
- o Stating areas where dogs have to be kept on a lead
- o Stating areas where dogs have to be put on a lead if asked to do so
- o Multiple dog walking in certain areas
- Dog Control Orders can be put in place by local authorities or parish councils. If an order is broken, then a fine of up to £1000 can be issued.
- Dog Control Orders in place for certain areas can be requested from the relevant local authority.

Protection of Animals (Anaesthetics) Act 1954, amended 1982

- This act serves to protect animals in making any operation at will cause pain without providing anaesthetic to relieve the pain, particularly if the operation involves sensitive tissue or bones.
- There are several exceptions to the act:
  - o Any procedure under the Cruelty to Animals Act 1876
  - o Emergency first aid situations
  - o Docking of a tail of a dog before its eyes are open
  - o Removal of dewclaws in a dog before its eyes are open
  - o Castration of a male animal before a specified age (details on the DEFRA website)
  - o Minor procedures usually carried out by a veterinary surgeon or nurse that is usually carried without anaesthetic as they are deemed to be painless
  - o Under permitted Home Office-licensed procedures
  - o The act does not apply to birds, fish or reptiles
  - o This act has been amended by the Welfare of Farmed Animals (England) Regulations 2007 (or other specified country, e.g. Scotland)

Veterinary Surgeons Act 1966, amended 1988 and 2002

- This act prohibits anyone other than a listed veterinary surgeon or listed veterinary nurse registered with the Royal College of Veterinary Surgeons (RCVS) from carrying out treatment or operations on animals. The exceptions are stated on Schedule 3 and are:
  - o Minor treatments given by the owner, household member or employee of the owner
  - o Medical treatments given to any animals used in agriculture by the owner, household member or employee of the owner
  - o Emergency first aid to maintain life and prevent suffering
  - o Castration or tail docking of lambs
  - o Removal of dewclaws in a dog before its eyes are open
  - o Anyone under 17 undergoing instruction in animal husbandry procedures either directly supervised by a veterinary surgeon or at a recognised institute of education under direct supervision

- The act also specifies certain procedures that can only be carried out by a veterinary surgeon.
- The Schedule 3 Amendment Order from 2002 states that only listed veterinary nurses who are registered with RCVS can administer medication under the direction of the veterinary surgeon. Student veterinary nurses can only administer medication under the direct supervision of a listed veterinary nurse or a veterinary surgeon.
- The Veterinary Surgeons Act is due to be reformed after consultation in 2012.

Welfare of Animals (Transport) (England) Order 2006

- This act replaces the previous transport-related legislation and falls under the directive of the Animal Health Act 1981.
- This order covers all vertebrate animals and also all cold-blooded invertebrate animals.
- The order makes it an offence to transport any animal in a way which causes or is likely to cause injury or suffering to the animal.
- Transport methods must consider space, ventilation, temperature and security of the animal, oxygen supply and liquid provision appropriate for the animal being transported.
- The order operates alongside a number of council directives which should be referred to prior to a journey occurring.

The Wildlife and Countryside Acts 1981 and 1985

- These acts replace several existing laws and regulations and cover the protection and conservation of wild animals and their habitats. Land, sea and airborne species of wild animals are protected. The minister can add to or remove from this list, species which may not legally be injured, killed or taken from the wild.
- The act protects habitats from humans and species in captivity which, if released into the wild, would seriously affect many other species.
- The act brings together and amends existing national legislation and EU directives covering protection of wildlife in the countryside, national parks and other designated areas.
- There is specific reference which makes it an offence to intentionally:
  o Kill, injure or take any wild bird
  o Take, damage or destroy the nest of any wild bird while the nest is in use or under construction
  o Take or destroy the eggs of any wild bird
- Amendments are in operation relating to specific parts of the UK (e.g. Scotland, Northern Ireland).

Convention on International Trade in Endangered Species of Wild Fauna and Flora (CITES) 1973

- Convention on International Trade in Endangered Species of Wild Fauna and Flora (CITES) is also known as the Washington Convention.

- The treaty is an international agreement that aims to protect the world's endangered species of animals and plants by controlling their export and import on a worldwide scale. Animals in this category are:
  - Those that are threatened with extinction
  - Those likely to become so threatened
- The treaty is voluntarily signed by countries who then agree to follow a framework to ensure that the CITES guidelines operate at a domestic level within that country. At the current time (2012), there are 177 countries that are signed up to CITES.

Animal welfare organisations

There are a large number and wide variety of animal welfare organisations in existence both in the UK and internationally that represent the interests of animals. These organisations may be specifically interested in the welfare of all animals or specific animals only.

The interests can be widely grouped under the following headings:

- Sport
- Conservation
- Health and welfare
- Registration bodies

Due to the sheer volume of animal welfare organisations in existence, examples can be provided, but there are too many to describe their work and do sufficient justice to them.

Examples of national/international organisations relating to each area can be found in Table 6.1.

Table 6.1   Animal welfare organizations.

Health and welfare	Conservation	Sport	Registration bodies
Royal Society for the Protection of Animals	RSPB	British Field Sports Society	The Kennel Club
Blue Cross	National Trust	The League Against Cruel Sports	Governing Council for the Cat Fancy
Dogs Trust	RBST	British Horse Society	British Rabbit Council
People's Dispensary for Sick Animals	County Wildlife Trusts	The Kennel Club	Weatherbys
The Donkey Sanctuary	World Wildlife Fund	Countryside Alliance	RBST
Animal Health Trust	International Union for the Conservation of Nature		
British Veterinary Association	European Association of Zoos and Aquaria		
Universities Fund for Animal Welfare	National Parks		
International League for the Protection of Horses	Flora and Fauna International		

Information about varying organisations can usually be acquired by either contacting the organisation directly or by looking at their website.

Animal rights

This term relates to a concept whereby animals should be entitled to the same considerations as human beings, and it is wrong to use them otherwise, for example, in recreational practices such as racing sports, in fishing, in hunting, in product testing and also as part of production processes.

Many people support animal rights and choose not to buy certain products, eat certain foods or attend certain sporting events. Some parts of society will actively demonstrate against such activities involving animals as they believe them to be cruel and unethical and these people are known as activists and they will freely call for the abolition of such animal activities.

The issue of animal rights will always be an emotive one, but it is generally agreed that animals do have rights; it is simply a question of what rights they have and to what extent these rights are invoked.

Chapter 7
Basic Animal Health Care

Summary

In this chapter, the learning outcomes are:

- To identify how to assess an animal's health status through the use of:
  - Behavioural indicators
  - Physical indicators including signs of pain
  - Physiological indicators
- To identify signs of health and suggest appropriate health routines
- To investigate factors that affect the health status of an animal
- To identify prophylactic treatments for animals including vaccinations, parasite treatments and microchipping

An animal relies on its owners/carers/handlers to regularly check its health and provide any necessary treatments when needed. Only they will know what is normal for that animal. In order to ensure that three of the five animal needs (see chapter 6) are being met, then it is ideal to keep all animals in the best possible health. Early identification of potential health issues can prevent more serious problems from developing later in the animal's life.

Basic animal health care refers to the routine observations that are carried out by the owner/carer/handler in order to assess the health status of the animal. Some assessments of the animal's health need to be carried out more frequently than others, and therefore, different routines can be put into operation according to the frequency of checks required.

Assessing the health status of an animal

When assessing the health status in animals, there are three types of indicators that can be used to obtain a complete picture of the health status of an animal:

Animal Biology and Care, Third Edition. Sue Dallas and Emily Jewell.
© 2014 John Wiley & Sons, Ltd. Published 2014 by John Wiley & Sons, Ltd.
Companion Website: www.wiley.com/go/dallas/animal-biology-care

- Behavioural indicators
- Physical indicators
- Physiological indicators

Behavioural indicators

Behavioural change in an animal is often the first sign that there is a problem. It is important whether there are any changes from the 'norm' for the animal being assessed.

Consider whether the animals:

- Are withdrawn
- Are non-communicative
- Appear fearful
- Appear to be in pain
- Are being actively aggressive
- Are not showing any change at all

Some animals (e.g. prey species) are very good at hiding when they are in pain, and so, behavioural indicators should not be the only type of indicator used to assess an animal's health status.

Physical indicators

Once the behaviour of the animal has been assessed, a full health check should be performed, as this will provide a clearer picture of the situation.

As well as performing a full health check (see later in the chapter), it is important to note the changes in the following:

- Posture and locomotion – is the animal moving normally?
- Feeding habits – has appetite increased or decreased or is the animal vomiting?
- Drinking habits – has water consumption increased or decreased?
- Toileting habits – is the animal toileting more or less often? What is the nature of the faeces produced? What is the colour of the urine produced?

Signs of pain

Signs of pain in an animal can include the following, but it will depend on the species of animal:

- Crying/whimpering
- Unusual body position, e.g. curled up
- The pupils of the eye are dilated
- Panting and heart rate are rapid
- Raised body temperature
- Not eating or drinking
- Unwilling to move or exercise

Physiological indicators

Physiological indicators give a more representative picture of what is happening within the animal's body. Detailed physiological assessment can only be carried out by veterinary professionals, but physiological indicators that can be checked by owners are:

- Temperature – is it raised or is it lower than normal?
- Pulse rate – check pulse rate, regularity and strength.
- Respiration rate – check respiration rate, depth and regularity. Note that one respiration is a single inspiration and expiration of air.

Combined together, this assessment is known as the **TPR assessment**. TPR assessments should only be done when the animal is resting but not sleeping and not straight after exercising.

Signs of health in animals

For these purposes, a dog will be used, but the same health check process can be used in all species although some slight modification may be needed depending on species. The health check should always be started at the head of the animal and finish at the rear end. An animal should be accustomed to this routine as early in life as possible as it means that examinations at a later age are easier because the animal is more tolerant and therefore the risk of any injury to the handler or animal is reduced.

Areas that should be checked on an animal when performing a full health check are shown in Fig. 7.1. Signs of good and poor health are shown in Table 7.1.

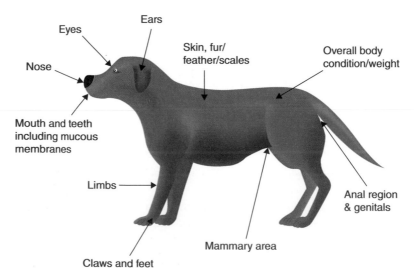

Fig. 7.1 Areas to assess for a health check.

It is also important to check:

- Posture, locomotion and gait
- Temperature, pulse and respiration rate

What is being looked for in each area?

Suggested health routines

Having an identified health routine makes it easier for owners/carers/handlers of animals to notice more quickly if there is a problem. Suggested checks are listed in Table 7.2, but routines will differ according to the species, age and existing health status of the animals.

It is worth noting that if an animal has an existing medical condition, is on treatment, is pregnant or is elderly, then your veterinary practice can guide you on the frequency of veterinary checks required. Working together with your veterinary practice promotes the best possible care for your animal(s). For animal collections, veterinary staff may assist in the creation of a health plan which ensures that health can be tracked across the collection and routine treatments planned for the best time across the year. Any changes to the existing health of an animal should be recorded and monitored, with veterinary assistance sought if necessary.

Table 7.1 Signs of good and poor health.

Area of the body	Signs of good health	Signs of poor health
Eyes	Clear and bright	Dull, cloudy, discharge, redness, swelling
Ears	Odourless, healthy colour	Excessive wax, discharge, redness, swelling, matted hair, cuts
Nose	Normal for species	Swelling, soreness, nasal discharge, crusting, abnormal for species
Mouth and teeth	Mouth, teeth and gums intact, healthy colour, good capillary refill time for mucous membranes	Soreness of mouth, swelling, broken teeth, blueness of mucous membranes, bleeding gums, signs of vomiting, offensive odour
Skin, fur/ feathers/ scales	Shiny, glossy, good condition of coat/feathers/scales, healthy colour to skin	Dull looking, matted coat, broken feathers, damaged scales, scratching, parasites present, soreness of skin, lumps, bumps, etc.
Overall body condition	Good body coverage, appropriate weight for the animal and its age	Excess or limited body coverage, obese or anorexic for the animal and its age
Limbs	Ease of movement, no swelling or obvious injury	Difficult or reluctance to move limbs, obvious injury, swelling, hot to touch

Table 7.2 Suggested health routines.

Daily checks	Weekly checks	Monthly checks	6 monthly checks	Annual checks
Food and water consumption	Coat and skin condition	Check nail length	Seasonal requirements, e.g. changes to housing or moving location	Annual vaccinations
Urine output	Ears for odour and wax	Check beak length in birds and chelonian	Parasite control – may be quarterly depending on product used	Veterinary health check – this may or may not include blood samples
Faecal output	Mouth, teeth and gums (Fig. 7.2)	Tooth length, e.g. rabbits and equids	Vaccinations, e.g. kennel cough, clostridial vaccine	Insurance if appropriate
Tolerance to exercise	Feel for lumps and bumps over the body	Overall weight and body condition		
General behaviour and temperament	Genital area for discharges			

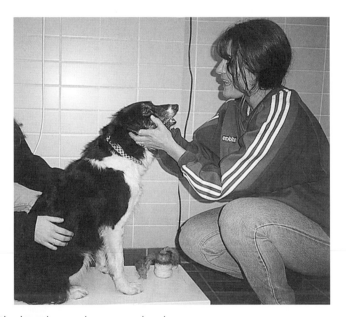

Fig. 7.2 Checking the mouth, gums and teeth.

Factors affecting health status

Many factors can affect the health status of an animal. Such factors may be animal related (Fig. 7.3) or non-animal related (Fig. 7.4). It is important to recognise that certain changes in an animal or its environment can affect the health status of the animal.

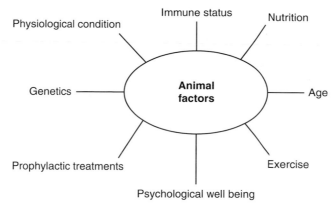

Fig. 7.3 Animal factors affecting health status.

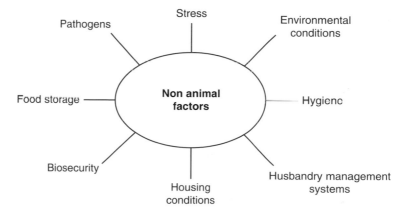

Fig. 7.4 Non-animal factors affecting health status.

Hygiene

Good hygiene is essential when dealing with animals to remove a build of pathogens from the environment which can otherwise cause illness in the animal. Again, splitting tasks into specific routines can help keep on top of things and minimise the risk of illness developing. The list in Table 7.3 is suggestions; routines will vary according to species and housing.

Exercise provision

Exercise is essential to animal health. Each animal has its own specific exercise needs, and an owner/carer should endeavour to meet these needs in order to maintain good welfare in the animal. When choosing an animal, it is important to consider the exercise requirements for the animal and decide whether these can be accommodated into your lifestyle. Many pets, dogs specifically, are abandoned and/or rehomed because

Table 7.3 Suggested hygiene routines.

Daily tasks	Weekly tasks
Wash food and water bowls/containers	Wash bedding
Remove "normal" discharges from eyes, nose, prepuce/vulva	Wash nylon harness or collars
Check coat/feather condition, groom as required (Figs. 7.5 and 7.6)	Groom thoroughly
Check anus for faecal material on coat	Disinfect grooming equipment
Remove faeces from environment	Disinfect housing
Remove any urine-soaked bedding	
Spot clean where necessary	

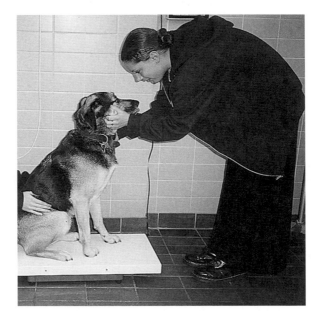

Fig. 7.5 Check coat condition.

people cannot meet their exercise needs. The frustrations on behalf of the animal(s) then tend to manifest themselves as destructive or unwanted behaviours. For example, a breed such as the Border Collie has a high requirement for exercise, whereas a breed like the Pug has a much lower one. Breed books clearly state requirements for exercise, temperament and suitability for potential owners. Life stages and life span will affect exercise needs.

Plenty of exercise is necessary for animals used in the areas of:

- Working (including uniformed work and also breeding)
- Racing

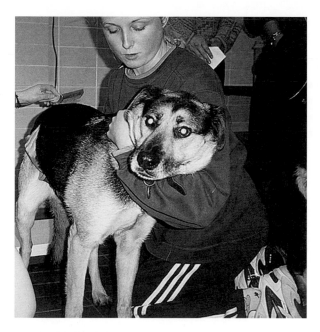

Fig. 7.6 Groom out the dead hair.

- Performance
- Agility
- Field trials

Less exercise is required for:

- Elderly animals
- Short-nosed breeds (brachycephalic)
- Some small breeds
- Animals with joint disease
- Animals with breathing and heart conditions

Some animals tend to 'self-exercise' but can be trained to walk on a lead, e.g. cats, ferrets and rabbits. Small pets will exercise if they have enhanced living areas with obstacles for climbing, toys and run areas, plus handling time, e.g. hamsters, guinea pigs and rats.

Companionship

An important aspect of health care is time spent in the company of the animal. Owners, carers and handlers can use this time to run health status checks. Dogs and cats are companion animals, and so, time must be spent with them to enhance their well-being – this also benefits human well-being. Some animals will respond badly to isolation, and this can be seen in their behaviour. Some breeds of cat and dog can suffer from separation anxiety, and all steps should be taken to reduce the amount of time that they are spent alone where possible.

Signs of isolation response include:

- Temperament change
- Destruction of housing
- Being aggressive or withdrawn
- Fear

Of course, in some cases, the earlier list could perfectly describe the normal behaviour of an individual. The only way to know if an animal is suffering from isolation response is to recognise what is normal for each individual, whatever the species.

Prophylactic treatments

Prophylaxis is the term given to a treatment designed to prevent the occurrence of a disease.

Vaccination

Vaccinations are treatments that are given to animals as a method of protecting them against potentially lethal disease(s).

Vaccines temporarily stimulate the immune system of the body and cause an immune response to the agent within the vaccine. The period of protection will vary depending on the species involved, the vaccine type and the individual receiving the vaccine. It ranges in most cases from 6 months to 1 year, at which point the animal must receive a booster vaccination to protect it further. The owner/carer/handler of the animal should know which vaccinations their animal(s) requires and how frequently they should receive them. If unsure, advice must be sought from the veterinary surgeon.

Parasite treatments

Parasites may be internal or external and treatments vary accordingly. Treatment of internal parasites is often referred to as 'worming', and the most common external parasites to be treated are fleas and ticks. Again, an owner/carer should have knowledge of what treatments their animal(s) requires and the frequency of application.

Microchipping

In February 2012, the government announced that from April 2016, all dog owners in England must have their animal microchipped in an attempt to reduce the number of strays and promote return of lost pets to their owners. This is also the case in Northern Ireland, but no plans are confirmed in relation to this in Wales or Scotland.

A microchip is a small electronic device, each containing a unique code. The chip is inserted through a needle into the most appropriate place on the animal for long-term existence and easy detection. In cats and dogs, this tends to be in the scruff. In bird species, it could be in the breast area, and in tortoises, for example, it may be implanted into the shell. The code is then logged with a registering organisation (e.g. Petlog), and the details are held on a database.

If a missing/stray animal is found, then many organisations (e.g. Dogs Trust, Blue Cross, PDSA, RSPCA), veterinary practices and dog wardens now scan the animal to see if it has been microchipped. It is hoped that compulsory microchipping will help reunite missing pets with their owners, but this relies on the owners keeping the registration information updated. Microchipping must be considered to be an essential and routine part of responsible pet ownership in the same way that vaccination and parasite treatments are.

Chapter 8
Disease Transmission and Control

Summary

In this chapter, the learning outcomes are:

- To identify the different methods of disease transmission including:
  - o   Vertical
  - o   Horizontal
  - o   Direct
  - o   Indirect – fomites and vectors (mechanical and biological)
- To identify disease transmission routes
- To identify methods of disease control
- To describe different methods of diagnosing disease
- To identify and describe types of basic animal treatments and their routes of administration

Disease is spread from one animal to another in different ways. The method and speed of transmission vary according to the type of micro-organism that causes the disease.

How can disease be transmitted?

When trying to identify how a disease is being spread between animals, the following questions need to be asked:

- How does the infection leave the infected animal?
- How is the infection passed from one animal to another?
- How does the infection gain entry to a new host?

Disease transmission may be described as being:

- Vertical
- Horizontal

Animal Biology and Care, Third Edition. Sue Dallas and Emily Jewell.
© 2014 John Wiley & Sons, Ltd. Published 2014 by John Wiley & Sons, Ltd.
Companion Website: www.wiley.com/go/dallas/animal-biology-care

- Direct
- Indirect

Vertical transmission

Vertical transmission occurs in pregnant animals when disease is passed from a dam to her offspring while they are still *in utero*.

The effects on the offspring depend on the stage of pregnancy, e.g. if a pregnant queen becomes infected with 'feline parvovirus', then the effects can vary from abortion in early pregnancy to cerebellar hypoplasia later in pregnancy.

Horizontal transmission

Horizontal transmission may occur due to direct or indirect contact.

Transmission through direct contact

Transmission of infection by direct contact includes:

- Contact between one animal and another, e.g. through grooming, fighting, greeting, mating (venereally), biting and being housed together
- Airborne over short distances, i.e. by aerosol infection also known as droplet infection, e.g. sneezing and coughing

The infectious agents that are spread by direct contact are often very fragile and cannot survive in the environment for long periods of time. Due to this characteristic, they are easily destroyed by light, heat and disinfectants.

Indirect contact

Transmission of infection by indirect contact occurs when:

- Two or more animals are in contact with the same inanimate object – the time between periods of contact by the two animals may be long, e.g. ringworm – which can remain viable in the environment for long periods of time. Common contact points are food bowls and water bowls, bedding and parks.
- Two or more animals are in contact with the same animate object.

For indirect contact to occur, the organism must be able to survive away from the host for a period of time. These organisms tend to be hardy organisms, and some are not easily destroyed, e.g. anthrax.

Transmission of infection by indirect contact is via:

- Inanimate objects – fomites
- Animate objects – vectors

Vectors may be mechanical or biological.

Mechanical vectors A mechanical vector simply acts as a moving fomite as the infectious organism does not develop, but the disease is spread:

- e.g. insects carrying infectious agents on their mouthparts.
- e.g. paratenic hosts – must be eaten by the definitive host in order to pass on infection. The organism lives in the tissues without developing – *Toxoplasma gondii* larvae live in mice and only develop once a cat eats the mouse.

Biological vectors A biological vector acts as an intermediate host for the infectious organism, and some part of the organism's life cycle occurs in the biological vector; therefore, the vector is essential to complete the life cycle of the organism:

- e.g. fleas, rabbits and sheep act as intermediate hosts in the life cycle of various tapeworms.

How does disease enter the animal?

Routes by which disease-causing organisms may **enter** an animal are shown in Fig. 8.1.

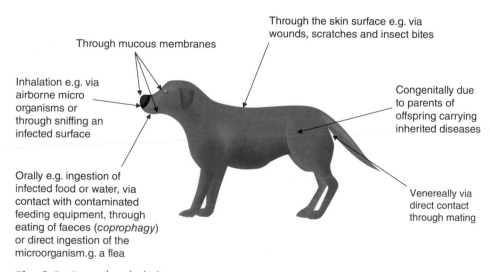

Fig. 8.1 Routes by which disease-causing organisms may enter an animal.

How does disease leave the animal?

Routes by which disease-causing organisms may **leave** an animal are shown in Fig. 8.2.

It is important to realise that dead animals can also transmit disease; hence, why there is strict legislation about disposal of dead animals.

When disease-causing micro-organisms are transmitted between animals, the infection can be transmitted by a carrier animal rather than an obviously infected animal. Carrier animals do not show clinical signs of disease but are:

- Individuals that have had the disease and recovered, called *convalescent carriers*. These animals may not have fully excreted the micro-organism and may remain infected for life
- Individuals that never show clinical signs of the disease and are called *healthy carriers*

Both types of carrier animal will excrete the disease-carrying micro-organism into the environment, putting other animals at risk.

Carrier animals can also be classified as continuous excretors or intermittent excretors.

Continuous excretors

- Animals continuously excrete the infectious organism.
- Can infect animals at any time.
- Relatively easy to detect than intermittent excretors.

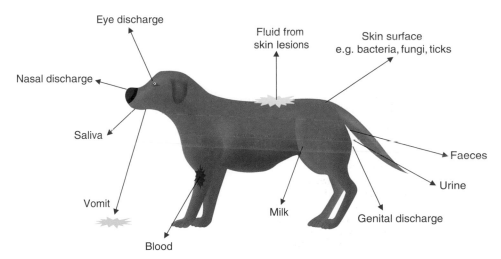

Fig. 8.2   Routes by which disease-causing organisms may leave an animal.

Intermittent excretors

- Animals that only shed the infectious organism at certain times, e.g. during stress
- May be shed during parturition, lactation, rehoming, weaning and when using steroid drugs

Incubation of disease

Incubation refers to the time between the host animal receiving the micro-organism and showing clinical signs of disease. The incubation period will depend on:

- *Number of micro-organisms received* – if received via the respiratory and/or digestive tracts, secretions here and movement of particles will prevent micro-organisms establishing, unless the animal is susceptible.
- *Immune status of the animal* – the animal may fail to mount an adequate immune response, allowing the micro-organisms to move on to their target tissues and establish themselves.
- *General health* – if not good, then the animal is susceptible.
- *Age* – the immune response of the body is reduced with age.

Infection

If the micro-organism has entered the host animal and overcome its resistance, infection is more than likely to be established. Some infections are confined to a restricted area and are known as *local infections*, e.g. abscesses; other infections spread through the whole body via the bloodstream and are known as *systemic infections*.

Resistance to infection

Individual resistance of an animal to disease will depend on:

- Age
- Nutritional state (too thin or overweight)
- Health status, e.g. no wounds on the body
- Vaccination status
- Immune response and white cell activity

Methods of disease control

- Avoid direct contact with infected animals (use of isolation).
- High levels of hygiene/disinfection in the animal's environment.
- Reduce the number of animals kept within the same airspace or improve the efficiency of air movement to reduce aerosol transmission.

- Provide early and effective treatment of infected animals to prevent others being infected.
- Control parasites to prevent passing of disease from one animal to another.
- Maintain vaccination status.

Infection terms

- *Subclinical* infection – has no clinical signs
- *Clinical* infection
- *Bacteraemia* – bacteria are present in the bloodstream
- *Viraemia* – viruses are present in the bloodstream
- *Pyaemia* – bacteria and white blood cells forming pus are in the blood
- *Septicaemia* – bacteria multiply in the bloodstream

Diagnosis of disease

Once it has been noted that an animal has signs of ill health by performing a full health check using physical and behavioural indicators, a veterinary surgeon will have arrived at a differential diagnosis. This is a list of possible diseases that the symptoms could indicate. In order to pinpoint the exact illness, there are a wide range of diagnostic tests that can be used to discover the underlying causes of disease and so begin appropriate treatment. Diagnostic techniques may be invasive or non-invasive:

- An invasive technique retrieves samples from the body cavity, e.g. tissue biopsies and blood samples.
- Non-invasive techniques retrieve samples without invading the body cavity, e.g. urine samples and faecal samples.

There are five major categories of tests for diagnosing illness in an animal:

(1) Biochemistry
(2) Haematology
(3) Bacteriology
(4) Urine sampling
(5) Faecal sampling

The test selected for use depends on the differential diagnosis reached by the veterinary surgeon and what is suspected as being the main underlying cause of the illness.

Haematology – involves taking blood samples from which a range of tests can be conducted. The blood is usually collected into a tube that is treated with an anticoagulant in order to stop the sample from clotting.

Bacteriology – identifies the bacteria causing a particular illness. Samples are taken from blood, mucus of skin scrapings which are then used to create a smear slide. Common strains of bacteria identified are *Staphylococci* (Gram-positive bacteria associated with skin and urinary infections) and *Escherichia coli* (Gram-negative bacteria associated with digestive upsets).

Biochemistry – involves the analysis of body fluid – usually blood, for products such as blood sugar, urea and creatinine.

Urine samples – urine can be collected from animals, and tests that can be performed on the urine include Clinistix tests where a stick is dipped in urine and a colour change occurs according to the type of problem, e.g. diabetes. If a bacterial infection is suspected, then the sediment of the urine can be made into a slide and examined in the same way as for bacteriology.

Faecal samples – examining faecal samples is very useful if trying to detect the presence of endoparasites such as roundworms and tapeworms by undertaking an egg count. Worm eggs look similar to grains of rice in the faeces. Faecal sampling can also be undertaken to establish if the animal is deficient in a number of enzymes.

Once the results have been obtained from the diagnostic tests carried out, then the veterinary surgeon can reach a final diagnosis and prescribe an appropriate course of treatment for the animal.

Basic animal treatments

Choice of medication

There are many different types of medication available to treat different problems in animals. The medicine chosen by the vet depends on:

- The part of the body the drug needs to target
- The speed at which the drug works
- The ability of the owner to give the drug

Types of medication

The sale and prescription of medications are strictly controlled to prevent misuse. The Medicines Act 1968 categorizes medicines according to the level of control needed over the drugs. Each drug is labelled with its category – see Chapter 23 for further information.

Routes of drug administration

The methods by which medicines are given to animals are called routes. Routes of administration for animals include:

- By mouth – orally (Fig. 8.3 and Table 8.1)
- On the body surface – topically (Fig. 8.4)
- By injection – parenterally

Oral administration

Medicines to be administered orally are given to the animal via its mouth.

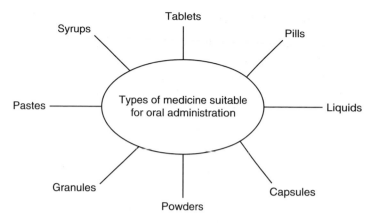

Fig. 8.3   Types of medicines suitable for oral administration.

Table 8.1   Methods of administering oral medication.

Type of oral medication	How to give to animal
Tablets Pills Capsules	• Directly to back of mouth or • Crushed in food
Liquids Syrups Powders Granules	• By syringe into side of mouth or • In drinking water • Mixed in food
Pastes	• Directly onto animal's tongue

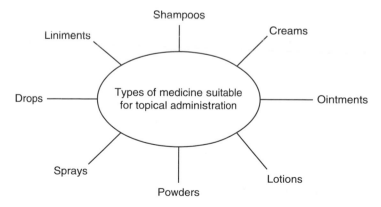

Fig. 8.4   Types of medicines suitable for topical administration.

Topical administration

Topical medicines may be applied directly to the skin or to the eyes and ears. How the product is applied depends on its type. Some topical medications need to be rubbed directly into the skin, some need to be dabbed on gently, some need to be sprayed on, and some need to be applied in drop form.

Parenteral administration

To administer an injection, you need a sterile syringe and a hypodermic needle of the correct size.

The most common routes of injection are:

- **Subcutaneous** – under the skin – usually in the scruff or loose skin on the back.
- **Intramuscular** – into a muscle – the muscle in the front of the hind leg is the most common site.
- **Intravenous** – into a vein – veins usually used are in the neck, foreleg and hind leg.

General guidelines when dealing with medicines

You must take notice of the instructions that come with the medication with regard to:

- How the medicine is to be applied
- How often the medicine is to be given
- Any special instructions, e.g. wear gloves
- The dose rate
- The expiry date
- The batch number

Medicines should be stored in a suitable labelled container and put away in a lockable cupboard out of reach of children and animals.

Records must be kept regarding all medicines given to animals in terms of name of animal, date of treatment, product treated with, expiry date, batch number, withdrawal period, etc.

Chapter 9
Basic Microbiology

Summary

In this chapter, the learning outcomes are:

- To identify the structure and function of:
  - Bacteria
  - Viruses
  - Fungi
  - Protozoa
- To identify and define basic terms relating to microbiology

Microbiology is the study and identification of micro-organisms (also known as microbes). The main micro-organisms to be considered are:

- Bacteria
- Viruses
- Fungi
- Protozoa

Micro-organisms are measured in micrometres or microns: *1 micron = 1 thousandth of a millimetre*. Microbes range from large protozoa to the virus, which is the smallest. Viruses can only be seen using an electron microscope and are measured in nanometres: *1 nanometre = 1 millionth of a millimetre*.
   Microbes are described according to their nutritional requirements:

- *Autotrophs* – synthesise (create) their own food
- *Heterotrophs* – obtain nutrients from their environment

Microbes live throughout the environment of humans and animals and are normally present on or within the body.

Animal Biology and Care, Third Edition. Sue Dallas and Emily Jewell.
© 2014 John Wiley & Sons, Ltd. Published 2014 by John Wiley & Sons, Ltd.
Companion Website: www.wiley.com/go/dallas/animal-biology-care

Microbial terms

- *Infection* – process by which microbes become established in the host.
- *Saprophytes* – live and feed on dead organic material.
- *Symbiosis* – the association between two different species living together.
- *Parasitic* – refers to the association between two different living organisms in which the parasite lives upon the host, taking food and shelter (host's own food or body fluids).
- Parasites fall into three groups:
  - (1) *pathogens* – will harm the host animal, causing disease
  - (2) *commensals* – will not harm but nor will they benefit the host
  - (3) *mutualistics* – are of benefit to the host, e.g. help break down food in the gut in some species.

Bacteria

Most bacteria range from 0.5 to 5 μm in length. They may be rod shaped (*bacillus*), round or spherical (*cocci*) or spiral shaped (*spirilli*) as shown in Fig. 9.1.

Structure of bacteria (Fig. 9.2)

- *Cell wall* – for shape and protection.
- *Capsule or loose slime layer* – for sticking to surfaces, protection from its environment and preventing destruction by phagocytic white blood cells.
- *Plasma membrane* – controls the passage of substances in and out of the cell.
- *Internal cell organelles* (cytoplasm, ribosomes, etc.) – to support the life of the cell.
- *Flagellum and pili* – hair-like structures for moving the cells along.

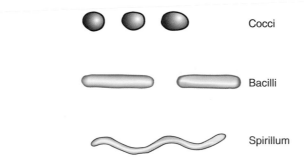

Cocci

Bacilli

Spirillum

Fig. 9.1   Shapes of bacteria.

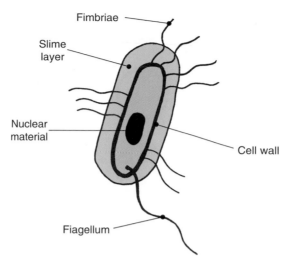

Fig. 9.2 Bacterium in detail.

Reproduction of bacteria

Bacterial reproduction takes place providing the following are available:

- Supply of nutrients
- Correct temperature
- Correct pH and oxygen levels, but it is important to note that not all bacteria require oxygen and are described as being *aerobic* or *anaerobic*:
  - Aerobic bacteria – grow in the presence of free oxygen
  - Anaerobic bacteria – only grow in the absence of free oxygen

Bacteria reproduce first by growth and then by division of the cell. Most reproduce by an asexual method called *binary fission*. For many bacteria, this division takes 15–20 minutes.

Binary fission

- One cell divides into two cells (Fig. 9.3).

Conjugation or bacterial mating

Sexual reproduction refers to the passing of genetic material and information from a bacterial donor to a recipient bacterium. It is passed through a short tube, the *sex pilus* (Fig. 9.4). This method passes part of the donor cell chromosome and extra genes, e.g. genes carrying antibiotic resistance factor, to another bacterium.

Some bacteria produce a dormant spore form (*endospore*). The production of spores is similar to binary fission, but the septum or divider is nearer one end of the cell and grows

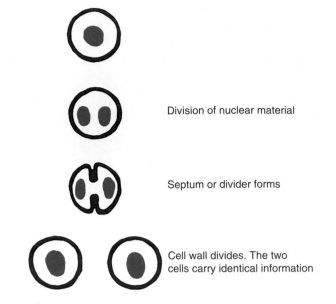

Division of nuclear material

Septum or divider forms

Cell wall divides. The two cells carry identical information

Fig. 9.3 Binary fission.

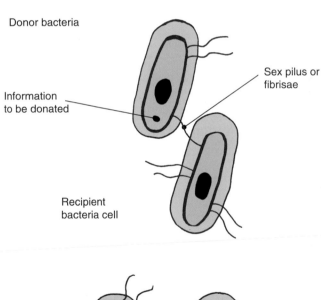

Donor bacteria

Sex pilus or fibrisae

Information to be donated

Recipient bacteria cell

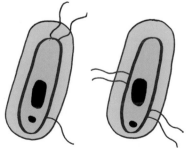

Recipient cell now has the 'passed' information

Fig. 9.4 Conjugation or bacterial mating.

to surround the genetic information. This creates a spore, the genetic information being contained within a protective coat or covering. This spore will form when conditions for life are not favourable, e.g. nutrients are not available. Once the spore forms, the original cell breaks down or *lyses*, releasing the spore into the environment to await improved conditions (Fig. 9.5). This is not a form of reproduction but a means of survival.

Bacterial terms

- *Endotoxins – toxins produced within the bacteria and only released into the host animal when the* bacteria die. The toxins can cause signs of shock or fever and can be lethal.
- *Exotoxins –* toxins secreted by the living bacteria which can also be harmful to the host animal's body.

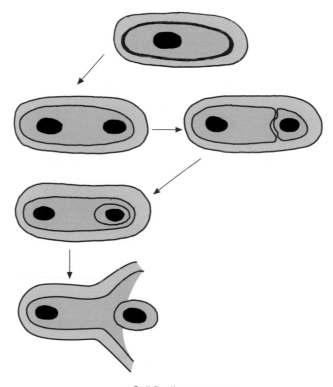

Cell finally ruptures to release spore which will remain in this form, protected, until its environment improves

Fig. 9.5 Spore formation.

Viruses

Viruses are the smallest of the micro-organisms (Fig. 9.6). They are always parasitic and reproduce by replicating themselves. This process happens after the viral DNA or RNA (genetic information) has entered a host animal's body cell. This strand of material takes over control of the host cell's metabolism and directs it to manufacture replicas of the viral material. When enough replicas have been produced, the virus will instruct the host cell to rupture, releasing the new viruses which go on to use other host cells for the purpose of replicating.

The virus is not a cell. In structure, it is a protein coat around a DNA or RNA strand. Some viruses are also surrounded by a membrane known as an *envelope* which may have structures like spikes on its surface for attaching to the host cell before entry.

In many cases, the cycle of viral infection causes no apparent harm to the host. Disease occurs when the host is harmed by the infection which occurs when quantities of host cells have been destroyed.

Fungi

These are non-chlorophyll-bearing plants, often called hyphae and divided into:

- *Moulds* – multicellular
- *Yeasts* – unicellular

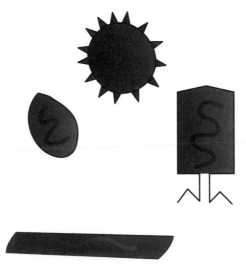

Shape variations with
DNA strand and protein coat
for protection

Fig. 9.6 Examples of virus shapes.

Table 9.1 Diseases produced by different microbes.

Microbe	Dog	Cat
Protozoa	Coccidiosis Toxoplasmosis	Coccidiosis Toxoplasmosis
Fungi	Ringworm	Ringworm
Bacteria	Kennel cough Leptospirosis	
Virus	Distemper Infectious hepatitis Parvovirus Rabies	Panleucopenia Respiratory disease Infectious peritonitis Leukaemia Immunodeficiency Rabies

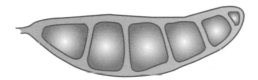

Spindle-shaped cells which make
up the spore, as seen in
Microsporum canis ringworm

Fig. 9.7 Fungal spore.

Fungi do not have the ability to create their own food and so must exist as parasites or saprophytes.

Distribution of fungal micro-organisms is by spores (Fig. 9.7).

Reproduction in fungi is sexual (hyphae from different strains unite into a survival spore form, awaiting favourable conditions), and there is also an asexual method (distribution of spores). Examples of diseases caused by fungi are ringworm and dermatophytes.

Protozoa

These are single-celled animals and range in size from microscopic to just visible to the naked eye. They have a cell membrane and have organelles for movement (flagella and cilia) (Fig. 9.8).

Reproduction is asexual by binary fission.

Nutrition is *holozoic* (capture and assimilation of organic material in their environment). Protozoa are capable of pursuing prey by following a chemical trail, or they can be stimulated by movement, particularly in water.

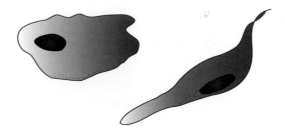

Fig. 9.8 Protozoa forms.

Protozoa will form a *cyst* at some point in their life cycle. This is the form which passes from host to host and allows temporary survival outside the host. Diseases caused by protozoa include toxoplasmosis and coccidiosis.

Chapter 10
Diseases of the Dog and Cat

Summary

In this chapter, the learning outcomes are:

- To identify and describe examples of diseases affecting dogs, covering cause, signs and treatments available
- To identify and describe examples of diseases affecting cats covering cause, signs and treatments available
- To identify types of immunity

It is important that owners/keepers of animals are aware of the diseases that may affect that animal but that the animal can be protected against. Vaccination is an important disease control method that can help to eradicate disease if the majority of animals are vaccinated against that disease.

Diseases of dogs

The infectious canine diseases for which dogs *should* be vaccinated against include:

- Canine distemper
- Canine viral hepatitis
- Canine leptospirosis
- Canine parvovirus

The infectious canine diseases that dogs *may* be vaccinated against include:

- Canine infectious tracheobronchitis (kennel cough syndrome) – optional but recommended if your dog visits a place where lots of other dogs visit, e.g. a park or a kennels (hence the name)
- Rabies – optional unless travelling abroad

Animal Biology and Care, Third Edition. Sue Dallas and Emily Jewell.
© 2014 John Wiley & Sons, Ltd. Published 2014 by John Wiley & Sons, Ltd.
Companion Website: www.wiley.com/go/dallas/animal-biology-care

Canine distemper

Canine distemper is caused by a virus that attacks the following body systems:

- Central nervous system
- Respiratory system
- Gastrointestinal system
- Skin

The disease is caused by a paramyxovirus that is closely related to the measles virus of humans. The virus is inactivated by light, heat and most disinfectants.

Distemper is most commonly seen in puppies of 4–5 months once they are no longer covered by maternal antibodies. Distemper has a seasonal occurrence in autumn and winter, due in part to the ability of the virus to survive in cold weather.

Routes of infection into a new host animal for the distemper virus are:

- Respiratory tract due to aerosol (airborne) exposure
- Mouth and eye mucous membranes

The incubation period of the distemper virus is 3–10 days, during which time the virus replicates and travels via the lymphatic system to the lymph nodes, spleen, thymus and bone marrow. Once in the lymph nodes, body temperature rises to between 39°C and 40°C for 2–4 days.

About half of all puppies infected with distemper are capable of mounting an adequate response and will produce antibodies to clear the infection at this point. If the virus continues, it replicates in the epithelium, organs and central nervous system. This allows secondary infection to occur.

Clinical signs of canine distemper include:

- Lack of appetite (*anorexia*)
- Nasal and eye discharge
- Coughing
- Diarrhoea and vomiting
- Hardening of the footpads
- Incoordination
- Paralysis
- Epileptic-type fits

If the puppy survives, the respiratory or gastrointestinal stage of the disease and the neurological signs develop up to 4 weeks later. Older dogs tend to present with just the neurological signs. Once neurological signs are displayed, the disease is usually fatal; occasionally, the dog will survive, but there will be lasting central nervous system damage.

Vaccination gives good protection but is not lifelong, so booster vaccinations are essential.

Canine viral hepatitis

Canine viral hepatitis is caused by the canine adenovirus type 1 (CAV1). It is a more serious disease in younger puppies than older dogs.

Transmission is through oral and nasal passages after exposure to infected materials.

The virus is highly resistant to destruction and survives outside the body for up to 11 days in bedding, feeding bowls, urine and faeces. It can resist freezing, ultraviolet light and most disinfectants but is destroyed by heat.

The incubation period for canine hepatitis is 5–9 days. Following exposure, the virus localises in the tonsils and lymph nodes of the animal where primary replication occurs. The virus travels in the lymph and gains access to the bloodstream. It is attracted to the cells of the liver and kidneys, where further replication occurs, before shedding occurs in urine and faeces.

Animals that recover from canine viral hepatitis can continue to shed the virus for several months subsequently; i.e. they are carriers of the disease.

Clinical signs of canine hepatitis include the following signs:

Puppies

- High temperature
- Death occurs within hours

Older dogs

- Survive the viraemic stage
- Bloodstained vomit and diarrhoea
- Acute abdominal pain
- In some dogs, 'blue eye', a clouding of the cornea of the eye, occurs up to 3 weeks after acute infection.

Vaccination and annual boosters are essential to protect dogs against this disease.

Leptospirosis

Leptospirosis is also known as Stuttgart disease or Weil's disease in humans; leptospirosis is caused by a filament-like bacterium, *Leptospira icterohaemorrhagiae*, which is a zoonotic disease.

A zoonotic disease is one that can be transmitted from animals to humans, and a number of precautions must be taken when dealing with animals that are infected with a zoonotic disease (see chapter 11).

The strains of the *Leptospira* bacteria that cause the disease in dogs are:

- *L. icterohaemorrhagiae* – (primary host is the rat) attacks mainly the liver
- *Leptospira canicola* – (primary host is the dog) attacks mainly the kidney

These bacteria are easily destroyed by sunlight, disinfectants and temperature extremes.

The disease is spread by direct contact, bite wounds or ingestion of infected food or water. Rodents such as rats are frequently carriers, shedding the bacteria in urine and thus contaminating water.

The incubation period for the leptospirosis is between 7 and 21 days, with severity of the disease caused depending on the susceptibility of the host animal and the strain.

Clinical signs of leptospirosis include:

- High temperature
- Shivering and muscle pain
- Vomiting and diarrhoea
- Dehydration
- Shock
- Jaundice (mucous membranes of mouth and eye appear yellow)

Animals that recover from *Leptospira* infection shed the bacteria via the urine for some time after recovery. Strict isolation procedures must be observed. Both veterinary surgeons and doctors can provide advice and information to prevent a human owner/keeper becoming infected.

An annual booster after initial vaccination is essential.

Canine parvovirus

Canine parvovirus is closely related to the feline panleucopenia virus. The virus is very resistant to inactivation by most disinfectants except bleach and formalin-based chemicals and can survive for months in the environment.

Following an incubation period of 5–10 days, the virus locates in lymphatic tissues and the intestinal epithelium lining. It is found in vast numbers in the faeces and vomit of infected animals and causes mild to severe haemorrhagic enteritis along with myocarditis.

The route of infection is by faecal or oral contact. Damage to the bone marrow results in lack of white cells, and the infection spreads from lymph cells in the gut tissues.

Clinical signs of canine parvovirus include:

- Being dull and depressed
- Anorexia
- High temperature (up to 41°C)
- Vomiting bloodstained gastric juice
- Bloodstained diarrhoea 24 hours later
- Becomes rapidly dehydrated

Vaccination as a puppy should be followed by annual boosters for ensured protection.

Canine infectious tracheobronchitis (kennel cough syndrome)

Kennel cough syndrome is a complex disease linked to a number of micro-organisms including a bacterium and a range of viruses:

- *Bordetella bronchiseptica*
- Canine adenovirus type 2 (CAV2)
- Canine parainfluenza virus (CPIV)
- Canine distemper virus (CDV)

The major primary cause is thought to be the bacteria *B. bronchiseptica*. Clinically, the syndrome presents as tracheitis, which is usually self-limiting but which may also develop into bronchitis or pneumonia.

B. bronchiseptica, CAV2 and CPIV are very contagious and commonly present when dogs are housed together, as they infect the respiratory tracts in dogs of any age. They cause nasal and tracheal inflammation lasting 5–14 days and then normally resolve, with the dog making a good recovery. At this time, the dog sheds the organisms in the respiratory secretions.

Clinical signs of CIV include:

- Cough
- Sneezing and nasal discharge
- Depressed but still eating
- Retching after coughing

Transmission from dog to dog is high in environments where there are a high number of dogs, and this is where the name kennel cough syndrome is derived from, but it is important to note that dogs do not just become infected from this disease in kennel environments. Risk of infection can be minimised by isolation of the affected animal and by improving the kennel ventilation and disinfection routines. All dogs that are going into a boarding establishment should have been vaccinated with a mixed vaccine that includes CAV2 and CPIV. Kennel cough vaccines may need to be re-administered every 6 months in order to maintain protection against the disease – it will depend on the brand of vaccination administered.

Rabies

Rabies is caused by a rhabdovirus. It is a fragile virus, surviving for only a short time in the environment, and is destroyed by most disinfectants, heat and light.

The rabies virus is transmitted in the saliva of infected animals. Following infection, the virus replicates in the muscle cells at the site of infection, from where it travels via the peripheral nerves to the spinal cord and the brain. Once located in the central nervous tissues, neurological signs of disease are observed. The virus also then travels to the salivary glands, where it is shed to infect other mammals, both human and animal. Rabies is a zoonotic disease.

The incubation period following infection is from 10 days to 4 months, depending on how near to the central nervous system the virus is initially placed. There are three phases or stages to the disease symptoms. However, not all stages will necessarily occur in all affected animals.

(1) *Preclinical stage* – lasting 2–3 days with a raised body temperature, slow eye reflexes and signs of irritation at the site of the original injury.

(2) *Excitable stage* – lasting up to 1 week with the animal becoming irritable, aggressive and disorientated, having difficulty standing and epileptic-type fits.

(3) *Dumb stage* – lasting 2–4 days during which the animal becomes progressively paralysed in the throat and skeletal muscles, leading to salivation, respiratory difficulties, coma and death.

In some cases, the preclinical stage can last for several months during which the virus is shed in the saliva.

A diagnosis of rabies is confirmed on postmortem examination of the brain and spinal cord for signs of the virus. A vaccine is available for dogs that live in countries where rabies is endemic or for travelling to a country with rabies in the wild or domestic animal population. The vaccine can only be given from 3 months of age, and boosters should be administered annually to maintain protection.

If a dog or human is bitten by an animal suspected of being infected with rabies:

- clean the wound immediately using soap or antiseptic solutions
- seek medical attention straight away

Other infectious diseases to be aware of are as follows.

Salmonellosis

Salmonellosis is caused by various strains of *Salmonella* bacteria. Salmonella infection is zoonotic. Salmonella bacteria naturally exist in mammals, reptiles and birds and are also shed in the faeces of these animals. Salmonella can exist in the environment for relatively long periods of time. Transmission from animal to animal or animal to human occurs when the bacteria are ingested via contaminated food or water or fomites in the environment. Younger animals and pregnant animals tend to be more susceptible to the disease. Overcrowding and stress can also increase the risk of salmonellosis. When nursing animals with *Salmonella* infection, barrier-nursing techniques must be adopted – see Chapter 21 for further information on this technique.

Escherichia coli: E. coli infection

There are several strains of *E. coli* in existence, but one of the most severe and dangerous infections is that caused by *E. coli 0157*. This strain can cause major digestive disturbance and is also zoonotic. In humans, it can cause kidney failure and death. *E. coli 0157* can be ingested from contaminated food or through contamination with the faeces of livestock that naturally carry the disease such as calves and birds. It is vital after undertaking any procedures with animals that hands are thoroughly washed and strict hygiene procedures are followed.

Diseases of cats

The infectious feline diseases for which cats *should* be vaccinated against include:

- Feline panleucopenia or feline infectious enteritis
- Feline viral respiratory diseases (cat flu):
  o feline herpesvirus
  o feline calicivirus
- Chlamydiosis or feline pneumonitis
- Feline infectious anaemia (FIA)
- Feline infectious peritonitis (FIP)

The infectious feline diseases that cats *may* be vaccinated against include:

- Feline leukaemia virus (FeLV)
- Feline immunodeficiency virus (FIV)
- Rabies (see Rabies in the dog)

Feline infectious enteritis

Feline infectious enteritis is a highly infectious disease of cats, also called:

- Feline parvovirus
- Feline distemper
- Feline panleucopenia

The disease is caused by a parvovirus, similar to canine parvovirus. The disease can affect cats of any age but is mainly responsible for deaths in young kittens.

The virus is stable and capable of surviving up to years in the environment and is resistant to most disinfectants. The incubation period is 5–9 days following direct contact with an infected animal, ingestion of the virus or through contact with objects used by an infected animal (fomites). The virus targets rapidly dividing cells and tissues of the small intestines, lymph and bone marrow. It is shed in saliva, vomit, faeces and urine for up to 6 weeks following infection. Cats can also be infected by dogs that may be shedding parvovirus. Kittens can be infected across the placenta in pregnant queens.

Clinical signs of feline infectious enteritis include:

- Diarrhoea, often bloodstained
- Dull and listless behaviour
- Abdominal pain
- Fever and dehydration

The virus can cross the placenta during pregnancy and affects the foetus by targeting the brain tissue (cerebellum), causing death or abnormal nervous system development.

Kittens show balance difficulties and incoordination at about 2–3 weeks of age if affected. If the cat survives the first week of clinical disease, careful nursing can lead to recovery, but the intestine may suffer permanent damage, seen as poor absorption of nutrients and constant diarrhoeal episodes.

Blood testing shows a reduction in white blood cells (leucopenia), particularly neutrophil white cells.

No specific treatment is available, and so, nursing treatment must occur in isolation as the disease is extremely contagious. Recovery is possible, depending upon the extent of the infection and how soon diagnosis occurs.

Vaccination using either live vaccine (or inactivated vaccine for pregnant cats) provides effective immunity with a booster every year. The term prevention is better than cure is highly applicable in the case of feline infectious enteritis.

Feline viral respiratory diseases

Many micro-organisms can be responsible for causing respiratory disease in cats, and the disease is complex.

Feline viral respiratory disease can also be known as:

- Cat flu
- Feline upper respiratory disease (FURD)
- Feline viral rhinotracheitis (FVR)
- Feline viral respiratory complex

The two main viruses involved are:

(1) Feline herpesvirus
(2) Feline calicivirus

Cats are particularly susceptible to infections (both bacterial and viral) of the nose and throat. Due to their location, these infections are called upper respiratory infections or cat flu. While it is essential to vaccinate, as with the 'human flu', vaccines do not protect against some strains of this disease, especially *feline calicivirus*.

Calicivirus is easily destroyed outside the host by disinfectants. Transmission of the virus is by aerosol or direct contact. As a result of this, any grouping of cats may lead to infection, i.e. shows, boarding, breeding kennels and veterinary surgeries.

Many cats that have survived the disease become carriers, shedding the virus for several years. It is possible to have suspected carrier animals tested by a veterinary surgeon for the presence of the calicivirus.

The incubation period is up to 10 days after exposure to high-risk situations (groups of cats) or stress caused by a change to the environment which may lower the cat's resistance to disease.

Clinical signs of calicivirus infection include:

- Ulcers on the tongue
- Inflammation of the gums

- Unwilling to eat but producing excess saliva
- High temperature
- Depressed and listless
- Loss of voice

The presence of ulcers may allow bacteria normally present in the environment to add to the cat's original symptoms and recovery time.

Feline herpesvirus can survive outside the host for up to 8 days. This virus attacks and replicates in the tissues of the respiratory tract and conjunctiva of the eye, causing viral rhinotracheitis. The tissues from the nose (*rhino*) to the trachea (*tracheitis*) are affected and inflamed, causing breathing difficulties, sneezing and coughing. Recovered animals can act as carriers, shedding the virus particularly when stressed.

Viral rhinotracheitis is the most serious form of upper respiratory disease, often leaving recovered animals with damage to the nasal passages. This causes the affected cat to periodically sneeze, snuffle and have a runny nose, the discharge occasionally being thick with pus.

The incubation period is from 2 to 10 days following exposure to the virus.

Clinical signs of feline herpes virus include:

- High temperature
- Discharge from the eyes and nose, later becoming thickened due to bacterial infection
- Depressed and listless
- Loss of appetite
- Sneezing
- Conjunctivitis
- Mouth ulcers
- Pneumonia
- Abortion in pregnant queens

Vaccination against both these viruses is available, and boosters should be given on an annual basis to maintain protection. In high-risk situations, 6 monthly administration is advisable.

Chlamydiosis or feline pneumonitis

Chlamydial infection is caused by an organism which lives within cells, and it can also contribute towards feline respiratory disease. Chlamydiae are therefore treated like a virus but in appearance resemble a bacterium. *Chlamydophila felis* affects the conjunctiva of the eye in cats, causing severe conjunctivitis with eye discharges, sneezing and nasal discharge. The conjunctivitis may affect one or both eyes.

Chlamydophila organisms are very fragile and cannot survive for any significant period of time in the environment. Infection therefore occurs through direct contact between animals.

Transmission is via direct contact between animals. The incubation period is 3–10 days.

Clinical signs of feline chlamydiosis infection include:

- Initial watery discharge in one eye, spreading to both
- Inflamed conjunctiva
- Signs of eye discomfort
- Fever
- In kittens, diarrhoea can also occur
- During pregnancy, chlamydia may cause abortion or stillbirth

Chlamydiosis may last for 2–3 weeks or longer, especially as a part of the feline viral respiratory disease complex. Recovered animals may shed the responsible organism for several weeks, so any treatment usually continues for 3 weeks following recovery. The organism is killed by most disinfectants during routine cleaning. Antibiotics are usually the primary treatment along with topical eye drops.

Vaccination is available against chlamydiosis with an annual booster required to maintain protection. It should be noted that the vaccine does not prevent infection but does prevent severe disease.

Feline infectious anaemia (FIA)

FIA is the direct loss of red blood cells caused by a group of bacterial parasites called haemoplasmas. Haemoplasmas live on the surface of the red blood cells, and the damage caused can subsequently cause anaemia to develop in the animal.

There are three main haemoplasmas that can cause FIA:

(1) *Mycoplasma haemofelis* – causes severe anaemia.
(2) *Candidatus Mycoplasma haemominutum* – causes mild infection often with no clinical signs observed.
(3) *Mycoplasma turicensis* – research is currently ongoing into the effect of this organism.

Transmission can occur through fighting and also from cats that are infected with fleas. Cats of all ages can be affected. When the disease is linked to feline leukaemia, white blood cell numbers are affected, and recovery of the animal is poor.

The micro-organisms responsible for FIA infection can be detected in a special blood smear examination in the laboratory or through a technique known as polymerase chain reaction (PCR) which serves to detect very small amounts of infection and also allows differentiation of the haemoplasmas.

The incubation period for FIA is up to 50 days, with recovered or carrier animals often shedding the parasite for the remainder of their life.

Antibiotics are used to treat the infection, and products to safely remove fleas from affected households are required, and other cats in the same household may need to be examined and treated. Further treatment may be required depending on the severity of infection. Your veterinary surgeon can advise on the most appropriate treatment plan.

Clinical signs of FIA include:

- Pale mucous membranes – mouth and gums
- Breathing difficulty
- Listless and loss of appetite
- Third eyelid up as a sign of ill health
- High temperature
- Weight loss

Currently, there is no preventative treatment for FIA.

Feline infectious peritonitis

FIP is caused by a feline coronavirus. Coronavirus is found in a cat's surrounding environment, and the rate of infection is especially high where many cats are found. Infected cats shed the virus in their faeces, and other cats can become infected via ingestion of the virus through eating or grooming, for example. Not all infected cats will develop FIP as the disease is only caused when the coronavirus mutates within the cat. The disease can be fatal.

Clinical signs include:

- Lack of appetite and gradual weight loss
- Lethargy
- Swollen abdomen due to an accumulation of yellow fluid
- Possible breathing difficulties dependent on amount of fluid in the abdomen
- Diarrhoea and vomiting

Progressive signs include:

- Neurological signs including inability to stand, paralysis and convulsions
- Inflammation within the structure of the eye, affecting sight

There are two forms of FIP. One form is characterised by the formation of fluid in the abdomen, and the disease is said to be 'wet' in form. If lesions form on the organs instead of fluid building up, then the disease is said to be 'dry' in form.

The disease can only usually be confirmed on postmortem examination as there is no definitive diagnostic test.

If clinical FIP becomes established, then the disease is fatal. Any treatment provided is to relieve suffering and alleviate the signs of disease displayed. Euthanasia should be considered if the disease is suspected.

In order to assist in preventing FIP, strict hygiene and disinfection are essential, particularly in multi-cat environments. There is currently no vaccine available in the UK to prevent FIP.

Feline leukaemia virus (FeLV)

FeLV is a common illness in cats caused by a retrovirus, and it affects approximately 1–2% of cats in the UK. Infection rates are higher in cats living in a multi-cat environment. The disease is contagious and, once symptoms appear, it is almost always fatal. Most cats are exposed to this virus during their life, and it is most commonly found where cats are in close contact.

FeLV is a fragile virus and cannot exist for a long time in the environment. Close contact between cats supports transmission of the virus. Transmission is via saliva either through fighting/biting, grooming or use of feeding bowls, water bowls, bedding etc. A pregnant queen may pass the infection on to her unborn young, or the virus can also be passed to kittens through milk in a lactating queen. Infected cats may become persistently infected, but this does not happen in all cases of infection.

Once the virus enters the body, usually via the mouth or nose, replication occurs before the virus enters the bloodstream. Once in the bloodstream, the virus targets the bone marrow specifically. Cats that can mount a suitable immune response to the virus will do so within 3 months, but if the bone marrow becomes significantly infected, then it is likely that the cat will subsequently suffer from a persistent infection. The virus is easily destroyed by disinfectants and cannot live long outside a host.

Commonly, the infection suppresses the immune system which then leaves the cat susceptible to infection from other diseases. Young kittens are most susceptible to the virus. Most die within 2–3 years of exposure or as a result of FeLV-related disease conditions, which include:

- Anaemia (lack of red blood cells)
- Lymphosarcoma (tumours of the lymph system)

Evidence of the virus' presence can be obtained through testing blood samples using several diagnostic tests.

Clinical signs of FeLV infection include:

- High temperature (fever)
- Lethargy
- Poor appetite and weight loss
- Anaemia
- Enlargement of the spleen

Control of FeLV disease is via:

- Testing, particularly in multi-cat households
- Animals testing positive being isolated from others
- Disinfection and strict hygiene in cat areas
- Retesting 12 weeks after positive test to ensure true result
- Testing all new cats that join a household

After two positive tests, the safe choice is to permanently isolate or euthanase the cat. Cats can be vaccinated from 9 weeks of age with a second dose 2–4 weeks later followed by an annual booster. Vaccination does not prevent FeLV infection, but it aims to prevent cats from becoming persistent shedders of the disease. Before vaccination, all cats are tested for presence of the virus in the blood.

Feline immunodeficiency virus (FIV)

FIV causes a worldwide disease of cats with approximately 6% of healthy cats being infected. FIV is caused by a virus of the lentivirus group. The disease is often characterised by a long incubation period. Incubation to signs of the disease can take from 4 weeks to several years; as a result of this, it is unusual to detect infection in cats under 2 years of age. The disease attacks the white blood cells which in turn affects and suppresses the immune system of the cat, leaving the cat more susceptible to other diseases. Initially, the disease was known as T-lymphotropic T cell lentivirus, due to the effect on the cells of the immune system (T cells and B cells).

The FIV is carried in the saliva of the infected animal and is most commonly transmitted by biting during fights. Therefore, cats that have access to outdoor life are more at risk than those housed completely indoors. Male cats are more commonly infected due to territorial fighting. The virus can also be passed on in cats that live in close social contact through grooming, sharing of food bowls, etc.

Commercial screening kits are available to detect antibodies to the virus from a blood sample. After the initial body response to the virus, the cat shows signs of the disease within a few weeks. These signs are very similar to those of FeLV and include:

- Conjunctivitis and nasal discharge
- Enlarged superficial lymph nodes (*lymphadenopathy*)
- Mouth and gum inflammation
- Diarrhoea
- Skin problems
- High temperature
- Neurological signs that include difficulty in walking and change in temperament

The animal then appears to recover, but due to gradual suppression of its immune responses, it will frequently suffer from recurring or ongoing infections of various kinds, often failing to respond to veterinary treatment. The cat will suffer weight loss, becoming inactive and listless.

There is currently no treatment to eliminate an established FIV infection. Any treatment given is to reduce suffering and alleviate the other signs displayed in order to promote a good quality of life.

There is no vaccine available in the UK, so owners are advised to castrate male cats and limit exposure to other neighbourhood cats in order to avoid contact with an infected animal. Cats known to be infected with FIV should be kept indoors.

Immunity

Immunity refers to the body's natural protection against life-threatening disease. It can be achieved by:

- Contracting the disease and recovering
- Vaccination

The purpose of a vaccination programme is to prevent the disease by preventing or limiting the infection in a host animal. Vaccines cause stimulation of the immune system which in turn produces *antibodies*. The cells of the immune system responsible for producing this protection are the B-lymphocytes, and these in turn are assisted by the T-lymphocytes. Both are white blood cells, which may be targeted and destroyed by certain viruses. The antibodies will recognise specific viruses or bacteria and prevent or limit their ability to produce disease in the host animal.

At the time of vaccination, the veterinary surgeon will fully examine the animal to ensure that adverse conditions which may influence the manner in which the body responds to the vaccine are not present, such as a high body temperature indicating infection.

There are many factors which influence an animal's ability to respond to vaccination. These include:

- Presence of colostral antibodies from the mother's milk which could interfere with the vaccine
- Vaccine type
- Route of administration – subcutaneous or intranasal
- Animal's age
- Medication that could interfere with the vaccine, i.e. anti-inflammatory drugs
- Diet
- Infection already present

Immunity may be acquired by passive or active means. Passive immunity results from the transfer of maternal antibodies to the newborn via the colostrum in the milk. The degree of immunity depends on the quantity of the first milk let down and the quality of the mother's own antibodies resulting from her recent vaccinations. Passive immunity lasts only as long as the antibodies remain active in the blood, from 3 to 12 weeks. After this time, the body will eliminate the antibodies.

Active immunity develops either as a result of the animal becoming infected with a micro-organism, developing the disease and recovering or from a vaccination. Both cause the body to react in much the same manner by stimulating the production of antibodies which are specific to particular microbes (*pathogens* or *antigens*).

Vaccines are prepared from live or inactivated (killed) preparations of micro-organisms. They stimulate the immune system of the vaccinated animal to produce antibodies to specific disease-producing materials.

Chapter 11
Zoonotic Diseases

Summary

In this chapter, the learning outcomes are:

- To define the term zoonoses
- To be able to name examples of zoonotic disease from a range of species
- To identify methods for preventing zoonotic disease

Also known as zoonoses or zoonones, these diseases are transmissible from animals to people. Most domestic animals can transmit zoonotic disease.

Dogs

Dog infection	Disease caused in humans
Leptospirosis	Weil's disease
Toxocariasis	Visceral larval migrans
Echinococcosis	Hydatid disease
Sarcoptic mange	Skin rash and bites
Cheyletiella mites	Skin rash and bites
Ringworm	Skin lesions and hair loss
Salmonellosis	Diarrhoea/vomiting
Rabies	Rabies (hydrophobia)

Animal Biology and Care, Third Edition. Sue Dallas and Emily Jewell.
© 2014 John Wiley & Sons, Ltd. Published 2014 by John Wiley & Sons, Ltd.
Companion Website: www.wiley.com/go/dallas/animal-biology-care

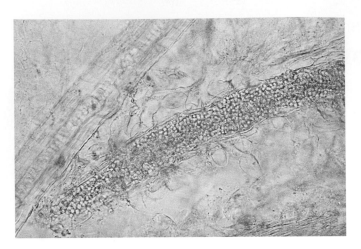

Fig. 11.1   Ringworm spores on a hair shaft.

Cats

Human disease	Signs in humans
Pasteurellosis	Bites or scratches become infected
Cat scratch fever	High temperature, flu-like signs, rash
Ringworm (Fig. 11.1)	Raised, circular, inflamed skin lesion
Toxoplasmosis	Abortion of foetus
Rabies	Fever, itching at original bite area, behaviour changes, paralysis and death

Zoonotic diseases from other species

Disease	Causal microorganism	Originating species
Brucellosis	Bacteria	Cattle
Campylobacter	Bacteria	Hamsters
Psittacosis	Bacteria	Birds
Salmonellosis	Bacteria	Mice, rats and guinea pigs
Tetanus	Bacteria	Horses and other herbivores

Prevention of zoonotic diseases

In order to minimise the risk to people of diseases which can be passed by companion animals, the following simple but effective hygiene precautions must be taken:

- Investigate any signs of illness.
- Control fleas and worms.
- Vaccinate animals.
- Do not allow pets to lick children's faces.
- Wash hands after handling any animal.
- Do not feed pets from household plates or dishes.
- Use separate utensils for food preparation.
- Daily collection and safe disposal of faeces.
- Always wear gloves when handling body discharges.

Chapter 12
Parasitology

Summary

In this chapter, the learning outcomes are:

- To define the term parasite
- To be able to name and describe the effects of key external parasites for a range of species of animal
- To be able to name and describe the effects of key internal parasites for a range of species of animal

Parasitology is the study of parasitic organisms.

A *parasite* is an organism that lives in or on another living body. The parasite benefits by taking its nourishment from the host. Parasites can either be host specific or they can have a range of hosts. Parasites may live on the inside or outside of the animal body. An *endoparasite* lives on the inside of the body, and an *ectoparasite* lives on the external surface of the host's body.

The parasite feeds on the host but does not want to deliberately kill it, as this would destroy its food source. Some hosts may die as a result of the parasite's feeding activities or from toxins released by it.

In order to prevent disease or death of the host species, prophylactic control of parasites is important (see chapter 7). Routine control in equine and large animals is necessary to keep parasite numbers down. Control in small animals (dogs, cats, rabbits, etc.) aims to completely remove all parasites, whether internal or external. There are many easy-to-use and effective products for removing external parasites such as fleas and lice, with a residue effect which will last for varying periods of time. The products supplied for eliminating internal parasites are collectively called *anthelmintics* or wormers. Some worms are zoonotic, and so, their elimination from the animal is extremely important.

Animal Biology and Care, Third Edition. Sue Dallas and Emily Jewell.
© 2014 John Wiley & Sons, Ltd. Published 2014 by John Wiley & Sons, Ltd.
Companion Website: www.wiley.com/go/dallas/animal-biology-care

Parasitology terms

- *Transport host* – transports the parasite to the next host. No development takes place in the parasite
- *Paratenic host* – same as transport but the parasite must be eaten, in order to be excreted and passed on to the next host
- *Intermediate host* – some parasites must spend time on/in this host in order to develop to their next life cycle stage
- *Final host* – host in which the parasite completes its development
- *Permanent parasite* – develops through all life stages and lives on one host
- *Temporary parasites* – move from host to host
- *Endoparasite* – lives inside the host's body
- *Ectoparasite* – lives on the surface of the host's body

External parasites

Fleas

Flea infestations are one of the most common problems occurring in dogs and cats. It can be almost guaranteed that every cat and dog will be infested with fleas at some time during their life. It is adult fleas that cause the clinical problems seen in animals.

Fleas can cause severe problems on their own, or they can also act as vectors for other organisms. Problems caused directly by fleas include:

- Severe skin irritation
- Eczema
- Anaemia
- Flea allergy dermatitis

Fleas act as vectors for:

- *Yersinia pestis* – causes plague
- Rickettsias
- Tapeworms

Common flea species

(1) Human flea – *Pulex irritans* (human fleas may also affect dogs, cats and horses)
(2) Dog flea – *Ctenocephalides canis* (dog fleas may also affect humans and cats)
(3) Cat flea – *Ctenocephalides felis*
(4) Chicken flea – *Echidnophaga gallinacean* (chicken fleas may also be found on dogs, cats, humans, cattle and horses)

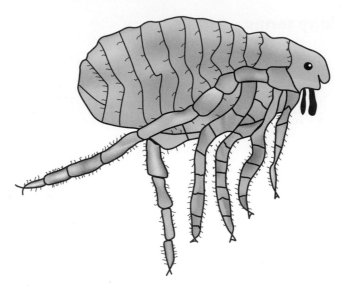

Fig. 12.1 Flea – *Ctenocephalides*.

Ctenocephalides species (Fig. 12.1)

- Adult fleas can live for 2 years without feeding
- Flea eggs hatch in 1–2 days
- Flea larvae feed for 4–8 days (in carpets or bedding)
- Larvae spin cocoons and adults emerge in 5 days or less
- Adult flea cycle may take only 3 weeks, but if the environment is unsuitable, the larval stage can last for months

Diagnosis of fleas

Fleas are often hard to detect due to their size. In heavy infestations, fleas may be seen in the coat especially in light-coloured animals, or they may have collected around the base of the tail, in the ears or in the groin/armpits.

The best and easiest way to check for fleas is to look for 'flea dirt'. Flea dirt is dried pieces of blood excreted by the flea. Comb your pet's coat over a piece of damp white paper or cotton wool. If the specks that fall onto the coat dissolve and turn red/brown, then your pet is likely to have fleas.

Prevention and treatment of fleas

A wide range of products are available for the control of fleas. It is important however to treat the environment as well as the animal. Products bought from the veterinary surgery are more effective than those bought from the pet shop:

- Sprays
- Powders
- Spot-on preparations

- Shampoo
- Pills
- Collars
- Liquid in the food

All products have their advantages and disadvantages – if you are unsure, seek help from your veterinary practice.

Ticks

Ticks are temporary parasites that spend short periods of time on the host, as they need more than one host to complete their life cycle. Ticks live on the surface of the animal's skin and feed on the blood of the animal. The ticks may produce toxins to aid with digestion. Ticks may act as vectors for microorganisms or endoparasites. When engorged with blood, ticks are easily spotted on the animal. Ticks may cause severe irritation according to their location and they may also cause alopecia.

Common species of ticks

There are three common types of ticks seen in animals and all are *Ixodes* species:

(1) *Ixodes ricinus* – sheep tick – very common and can affect various species
(2) *Ixodes hexagonus* – hedgehog tick – common and can affect various species
(3) *Ixodes canisuga* – dog tick – affects various species. Can be a problem in kennels as it can survive in crevices in floors and walls

Ixodes spp. (Fig. 12.2)

- Adult tick can live for 2 years without feeding
- Engorged female can lay 1000–3000 eggs
- Larva hatches in 30 days
- Nymphs emerge from moulted larva
- Adult tick emerges after 12 days
- Feeding is required between each stage of development

Diseases can be transmitted by ticks in their saliva to other host animals. These diseases include:

- Lyme disease – a bacterial tick-borne infection caused by *Borrelia burgdorferi*. The bacteria can cause skin discolouration along with cardiac and joint disease in the infected animal. It is endemic in a number of states in the USA. It is also carried in Europe by ticks of wildlife hosts, such as rodents and deer. Signs of Lyme disease are:
  o sudden onset of lameness with arthritic pain in one or more joints (i.e. carpal or wrist joint) which may last only a few days, recurring at intervals
  o high temperature with enlarged surface lymph nodes

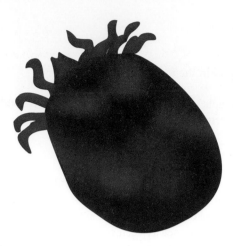

Fig. 12.2 Tick – *Ixodes*.

- Ehrlichiosis – caused by a parasite which lives inside certain white blood cells. It is transmitted by ticks during feeding on the host animal's blood. It is found in the Mediterranean basin in Europe and other Mediterranean countries. The severity and recovery of the host animal depend on the activity of its immune system. Certain breeds of dog are particularly susceptible to the disease, e.g. German shepherds. Babesiosis may also be present, having been passed by the tick at the same time. Signs of ehrlichiosis are:
    - high temperature and inappetence
    - lymph nodes enlarged
    - bleeding from the nose and under the skin
    - anaemia
- Babesiosis – caused by a protozoan that develops and multiplies in the salivary glands of the tick, from where it is transmitted to the host animal during feeding. It is endemic across much of Europe. The parasitic protozoa infect red blood cells. The severity of the disease varies, depending on the species and strain of *Babesia* and the health status of the infected animal. Signs of babesiosis are:
    - pale mucous membranes
    - anaemia
    - breathing problems and collapse

Treatment of ticks

- To remove a tick, dab with an acaride and remove with a specialist device. Surgical spirit may also be used but it is not always effective.
- Do not pull live ticks off as their mouthparts can be left embedded in the skin and so cause a secondary infection.
- Ivomec injections may also be given in animals where there is repeated and heavy tick infestation.

Lice

Lice are host-specific parasites. This means that they only live on one species, i.e. each animal species has its own type of louse. Lice can affect cats, dogs, rabbits, guinea pigs, rodents, birds and humans. Lice can be classified as biting or sucking lice depending on their feeding technique. They are transmitted either by direct contact or by eggs collected and passed on during grooming.

Problems that can be caused by lice

Lice can cause severe problems on their own, or they can also act as vectors for other organisms such as rickettsias.

Problems that may be caused directly by lice include:

- Severe irritation and pruritus.
- Loss of condition.
- Alopecia.
- Depression.
- Anaemia in severe sucking louse infestations.
- Excessive scratching due to lice can cause tissue damage and secondary infection.

Common species of lice

- *Trichodectes canis* – canine-biting louse
- *Trichodectes equi* – equine-biting louse
- *Linognathus setosus* – canine-sucking louse

The louse's life cycle

Lice complete their whole life cycle on the host by:

- Laying and cementing their eggs to the hair shafts. Louse eggs are commonly known as nits.
- Once hatched, the immature lice are identical to the adults except for their size and known as nymphs.
- After several moults, the immature lice become adults.
- The whole life cycle takes approximately 2–3 weeks.

Diagnosis and treatment of a louse infestation

Lice are often easily spotted due to their size.

A range of products are available for the control of lice. It is important however to treat the environment as well as the animal. Thoroughly disinfect the environment and replace any bedding with fresh, clean bedding. The animal may need to be washed in an insecticidal shampoo. If seen by a vet, the animal is likely to be given an Ivomec injection.

Mites

Mites either live on the surface of an animal's skin, or they tend to burrow just under the skin and so are classified as burrowing mites or surface mites. Mites are very small in size and can only just be seen by the naked eye.

Common species of mites

There are five common types of mites that affect animals:

(1)   *Sarcoptes* – burrows into skin
(2)   *Psoroptes* – bite surface
(3)   *Demodectes* – burrows into skin
(4)   *Otodectes* – live on surface
(5)   *Cheyletiella* – live on the surface

The mite's life cycle

Mites complete their whole life cycle on the host:

(1)   Females lay their eggs.
(2)   Eggs hatch into larvae.
(3)   Larvae undergo several moults to become adults.

A mite's life cycle can be as short as 13 days in some species.

Treatment of mites

Clean the infected area and use an acaricide to kill the mites. Repeat treatments are needed at regular intervals to ensure all life cycle stages are eliminated. Ivomec injections may also be given.

Sarcoptes mites (e.g. Sarcoptes scabiei)

- Burrow into skin surface
- Collect where there is little hair growth, i.e. around the ears, face, muzzle and elbows
- Presence of mites + intense scratching = soreness and damaged skin tissue
- Hair loss and possible secondary infection
- May get pustule formation
- Causes sarcoptic mange

Psoroptes mites

- Live on skin surface
- Cause localised lesions
- Live in the scabs formed by lesions from their bites

- Can cause sheep scab, body mange and ear mange
- e.g. *Psoroptes cuniculi* causes ear canker in rabbits

Demodectes *mites*

- Burrowing mites
- Found in dogs – *Demodex canis*
- Causes a non-itchy alopecia and skin thickening
- May spread to cause demodectic mange which may be dry or it may allow secondary bacterial infection to establish
- A similar mite is found in guinea pigs – *Trixacarus caviae*

Otodectes *mites*

- Surface mites living in the external ear canal.
- Causes irritation and can lead to intense head shaking and aural haematomas.
- Causes otitis.
- The most common type is *Otodectes cynotis*.

Fur mite: Cheyletiella species

Cheyletiella mites can be found all over the body surface. They live off the dead skin and carry it around the skin surface and so referred to as 'walking dandruff'. *Cheyletiella* mites cause an itchy dermatitis which is characterized by small red spots from the bites.

There are three main species of *Cheyletiella* mite seen in small animals:

(1) *Cheyletiella yasguri* – canine species
(2) *Cheyletiella blakei* – feline species
(3) *Cheyletiella parasitivorax* – rabbits and guinea pigs

Cheyletiella *life cycle*

- Eggs are laid and cemented to coat hairs, similarly to lice
- Eggs hatch into six-legged larvae
- Moult into eight-legged larvae
- Adult stage is reached

Cheyletiella mites are treatable with insecticidal shampoos.

It is important to note that *Cheyletiella* mites are zoonotic and also highly contagious. They can burrow through clothing and cause intense itching in humans. Adopt barrier-nursing techniques if possible.

Flies

Flies can also be parasitic to animals. Flies are attracted to soiled areas whether in the housing or on the animal itself. They lay their eggs, and once the maggots have hatched, they burrow into the skin of the animal, causing a condition known as fly strike.

Prevention of fly strike is particularly important in longer-haired animals, e.g. Angora rabbits, and also in livestock such as sheep. During hot, summer months, it is best to clip the rear end of species prone to fly strike to make detection of any soreness that may be caused by flies and maggots easier.

Ectoparasites in birds

Ectoparasites that can be seen in captive birds are described in this section.

Mites

Cnemidocoptes – mainly seen in budgies and canaries – causes scaly beak and feet. In pigeons, this species of mite causes feather disintegration.

Dermanyssus – red feather mite – seen in raptors, pigeons and parrots. This mite lives in the crevices of the housing and attacks the birds when they are roosting at night. As they suck the blood, this mite can cause anaemia.

Ornithonyssus – the northern fowl mite – this mite sucks the host's blood and lives on the host continuously, and so, it is easier to detect and treat.

Sarcoptes mites are not usually seen in birds but there have been recorded incidences in macaws.

Lice

All lice found on birds belong to the order *Mallophaga* and cause damage by chewing the feathers.

Lice are more common in birds housed outdoors due to transmission from wild bird species.

Flies

Many different families of flies can affect birds, e.g. blue, black and green bottles. Flies are attracted to birds with diarrhoea, they lay their eggs and the maggots eat into the bird and can cause a great deal of soreness in the rear area.

Ticks

Tick infestations can be rapidly fatal in birds due to a toxin in the saliva of the tick. Quite rare but can be seen in hunting raptors and birds kept in aviaries under trees.

Ectoparasites in reptiles

Ectoparasites that can be seen in reptiles are described in this section.

Mites

Ophionyssus natricis – this is the most commonly found mite in snakes and appears as red-dark pinhead mites living under the overlapping edges of scales. The mites may also be seen in water dishes after bathing has occurred. The mites can cause severe irritation and trauma as well as anaemia and dysecdysis (problems with skin shedding). These mites may also transmit *Aeromonas* spp. of bacteria and this can cause septicaemia in the animal.

Flies

Tortoises can suffer from fly infestations in the summer months if housed outdoors. The maggots can burrow into the tortoise within 2 hours and cause severe trauma, infection, shock and even death.

Ticks

Wild-caught reptiles often suffer from ticks but so may garden-kept tortoises. The ticks commonly seen in the UK are *I. ricinus and I. hexagonus*. These ticks may transmit the bacteria S*taphylococcus aureus* and *B. burgdorferi* that causes Lyme disease.

Internal parasites

Endoparasites for small animals are divided into two groups:

(1)   Roundworms (nematodes) (Fig. 12.3):
    (a)   are unsegmented
    (b)   have a body cavity
    (c)   have an alimentary tract throughout

Roundworms can be divided into six groups:

- Ascarids
- Hookworms
- Lungworms
- Whipworms
- Heartworms
- Bladder/liver worms

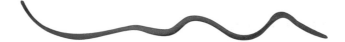

Fig. 12.3   Roundworm.

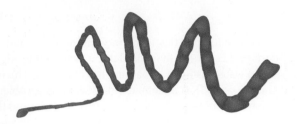

Fig. 12.4 Tapeworm.

(2)   Tapeworms (cestodes) (Fig. 12.4):
  (a)   are segmented
  (b)   each segment is independent
  (c)   have a complete alimentary tract in each segment

Animals infested with internal parasites do not always show signs of infestation. The signs only start to appear if the infestation becomes overwhelming to the health of the host animal:

- Scooting on bottom (anal irritation)
- Constantly hungry and eating (polyphagia)
- Weight loss
- Vomiting and diarrhoea seen in heavy infestation
- Unhealthy, dull coat
- Enlarged abdomen

Common worms in the UK include:

- Roundworms
  (a)   *Toxocara canis*
  (b)   *Toxocara cati*
- Tapeworms
  (a)   *Dipylidium caninum*
  (b)   *Echinococcus granulosus*
  (c)   *Taenia* species

Roundworms

Toxocara canis

This worm causes zoonotic disease. It can migrate in human tissues and is linked to a disease called 'visceral larval migrans' in humans, which can cause blindness in children.

(1)   Infective eggs or larval forms of this roundworm are swallowed by the dog
(2)   They migrate to the body tissues, often migrating to developing foetuses
(3)   They localise in the intestines, moving to the unborn before the end of pregnancy or infecting them through the mother's milk after birth
(4)   The larvae now mature, passing eggs in the puppies' faeces

(5)   These are swallowed by other puppies or the mother, and the cycle repeats unless the dogs are treated. Puppies should be wormed monthly from 3 weeks of age

Toxocara cati

This species of roundworm is responsible for infections in cats and kittens.

(1)   Kittens obtain the larvae of the tapeworm either from their mother's milk or from ingestion of eggs in the environment.
(2)   Adult cats gain the infection through ingestion of eggs in the environment or paratenic hosts.
(3)   Heavy infections lead to stunted growth and potbellied kittens. Kittens should be regularly wormed (monthly) from 3 weeks of age.

Prevention of toxocariasis

- Worm animals regularly
- Control the intermediate hosts (fleas and lice)
- Dispose of faeces immediately
- Disinfect where faeces have been
- Always wash hands thoroughly
- Wash animals' bowls separately from human utensils
- Do not let the animal lick your face
- Keep the animal's anal area clean
- Examine faeces regularly for signs of worms

Lungworms

Lungworms have increased in prevalence in recent years, and it is now recommended that dog owners particularly routinely worm their pets for lungworm:

- *Angiostrongylus vasorum* – dog lungworm
  Dogs become infected when they eats snails containing the infective larvae. These worms are very slender and live in the pulmonary artery of the dog. Signs of infection include irregular breathing and coughing.
- *Aelurostrongylus abstrusus* – cat lungworm
  Cats become infected by eating slugs and snails that contain the infective larvae. The adult worm lives in the cat's lung tissue, and a heavy burden may cause excessive coughing.

Hookworms

Hookworms have short, stout appearance with hooked heads. Two species may be found and they differ in the appearance of their head:

- *Uncinaria stenocephala* – plates in mouth – tends to affect greyhounds and dogs in hunt kennels and is found in the small intestine of dogs
- *Ancylostoma caninum* – large teeth – found in the small intestine of dogs

As their name suggests, hookworms attach to the small intestine with their mouthparts and use their teeth to damage the surface and then digest the damaged tissue. They can cause weight loss and anaemia. Their eggs are passed into the environment in faeces.

Whipworms

Whipworms, as their name suggests, have a whip-like appearance. The worms burrow into the large intestine to feed. The eggs are characteristic of the worm and are protected by a thick shell that makes them resistant to damage in the environment. They can survive in the ground for several years. Whipworms are rarely seen in the UK but an example is *Trichuris vulpis* – whipworm of the dog.

Heartworms – e.g. *Dirofilaria immitis*, heartworm of the dog – tends not to occur in the UK at the current time but may be seen in dogs imported from warmer countries.

Bladder/liver worms (*Capillaria* species) are not found in the UK at the current time.

Tapeworms

Dipylidium caninum

This tapeworm affects both dogs and cats and uses the flea as an intermediate host.

(1)   Animal passes egg-filled tapeworm segments in its faeces (Fig. 12.5)
(2)   The segments burst, releasing individual eggs that are eaten by the flea larvae
(3)   During grooming, the animal swallows the tapeworm-carrying flea larvae
(4)   The tapeworm matures in the animal host
(5)   The adult tapeworm releases mature, egg-filled segments

If the host is not treated with anthelmintic drugs, the cycle begins again and will continue to repeat to increase the level of infection.

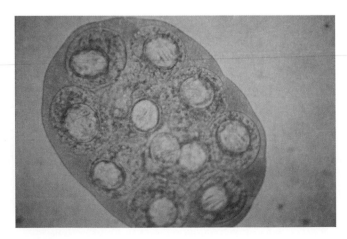

Fig. 12.5   *D. caninum* worm egg.

Echinococcus granulosus granulosus

This is an important **zoonotic** parasite in the UK. This parasite has a dog to sheep life cycle and so is found more commonly in rural areas. Adults of this species are approximately 6 mm in length, and there can be thousands in one animal's intestines. Treatment includes preventing access to sheep carcasses.

Zoonotic implications – if humans ingest an egg or a segment from their dog, then a cyst called a hydatid cyst may develop in their liver or their lungs in much the same way as it does in the sheep. Infected people are treated using an anthelmintic prior to drainage of the cyst. Surgical removal of the wall of the cyst is necessary and this can be hazardous to the patient.

Echinococcus granulosus equinus

This species has a dog to horse life cycle and is common in hounds fed on horse offal. This species is not believed to be zoonotic.

Tapeworms in other animals

Other species that may be infected with tapeworms include birds, rabbits, mice, rats and hamsters. All tapeworms are specific to a species and the intermediate hosts tend to be mites or beetles.

Treatment of tapeworms in general

Adult tapeworms are much easier to destroy than immature tapeworms. Treatment includes the use of an anthelmintic that has specific activity against a tapeworm (cestocidal). The product used may also have activity against roundworms and so may be called a broad-spectrum anthelmintic. More than one dose may be required if the infestation is heavy.

Chapter 13
Hygiene

Summary

In this chapter, the learning outcomes are:

- To explain the concept of hygiene and define other terms associated with this concept
- To be able to describe the properties, effectiveness, choice, types and use of disinfectants and antiseptics available
- To be able to explain the relevant health and safety related to the use of disinfectants and antiseptics
- To explain an ideal cleaning routine for animal housing
- To explain the use of alcohol gels in animal establishments

When working with animals, hygiene is of paramount importance with an aim to prevent the build-up of pathogenic microorganisms and the establishment of disease. Keeping the environment that an animal comes into contact with clean and hygienic contributes to reducing the chances of disease. Using disinfectants and antiseptics helps towards this aim.

Disinfectants and antiseptics

Disinfectants and antiseptics are chemical compounds that play an important role in maintaining the health and/or promoting the recovery of an animal. Their use in basic hygiene for housing, kennels, catteries or in veterinary practice hospitals is important to the care of both the environment and living tissues.

Disinfectants tend to be designed for use on the environment and non-living structures, including the furniture within an animal's housing, whereas antiseptics tend to be designed for use on living tissue. As both of these products are chemicals, if they are used incorrectly, such as at lower than advised concentrations, micro-organisms may develop resistance, thus reducing the value of the disinfectants and antiseptics to the maintenance of hygiene.

Animal Biology and Care, Third Edition. Sue Dallas and Emily Jewell.
© 2014 John Wiley & Sons, Ltd. Published 2014 by John Wiley & Sons, Ltd.
Companion Website: www.wiley.com/go/dallas/animal-biology-care

Terms relating to hygiene

- *Asepsis* – is a state of being free from micro-organisms.
- *Antisepsis* – preventing infection through use of antiseptics.
- *Disinfection* – the process of killing micro-organisms.
- *Sterilisation* – the removal or destruction of all living micro-organisms including bacterial spores. Always used on surgical instruments.
- *Cleaning* – the process of removing dirt (not necessarily micro-organisms).
- *Antiseptics* – chemicals that kill or prevent infection without damaging living tissue. They are referred to as *bacteriostatic*, i.e. they will prevent organisms from multiplying, and therefore, infections cannot develop. Can also be referred to as skin disinfectants as they are non-toxic and are applied to skin prior to operations or to broken skin to treats wounds or burns.
- *Disinfectants* – chemicals that kill microorganisms by either killing the organism or inhibiting its growth. Generally too toxic to be applied to living tissues and so are usually used on hard surfaces, equipment and instruments. Can be referred to as *bactericidal*, i.e. they will kill micro-organisms.
- *Bactericidal* – kills bacteria.
- *Virucidal* – kills viruses.
- *Fungicidal* – kills fungi.
- *Bacteriostatic* – inhibits growth of bacteria.
- *Fungistatic* – inhibits growth of fungi.
- *Virustatic* – inhibits growth of viruses.

Disinfectants

Disinfectants should only be used on the animal's environment, on surfaces such as floors, walls, ceilings, exercise runs and food bowls. Disinfectants are harmful to living tissues, and so, whenever disinfectants are being used, protective clothing should be worn – gloves, apron and face mask if working in an enclosed area. **Animals must always be removed from their enclosures when a disinfectant is being used**.

Properties of an ideal disinfectant

- Effective against a wide range of microorganisms
- Non-toxic to humans or animals
- Does not stain housing or clothing
- Is able to wet the surface being disinfected easily
- Penetrates through any organic matter on the surfaces being disinfected
- Is easily stored
- Can be stored for a long time (long shelf life)
- Only needs to be used in low concentrations for maximum effectiveness
- Cheap to use
- Readily available

Do disinfectants always work?

The activity of a disinfectant is affected by:

- The presence of organic matter such as faeces, blood and pus.
- Other chemicals being used at the same time, e.g. detergents or antiseptics.
- Type of water – hard or soft.
- Temperature of water – hot or cold.
- Time left on the surface.
- Material being disinfected can affect the efficiency of a disinfectant – e.g. cork, rubber, plastic, wood.
- The dilution rate of the disinfectant.
- The length of time the diluted product has been made up for.

Disinfectants are most effective when:

- Used with hot/warm water rather than cold.
- Left in contact with surfaces for the correct amount of time (see instructions on label).
- Used at the correct strength.
- Not mixed with other chemicals including soaps, detergents and other cleaning agents.
- Freshly prepared (see instructions on label).
- The amount needed is made up at any one time.

When choosing a disinfectant for the cleaning of housing and surfaces, careful choice is needed. Some products are toxic to certain species of animals. The phenols or phenol-containing compounds are toxic to cats, rabbits and rodents, so they tend to be used only in large animal and farming industry facilities. Products in this group are recognised as black, white or clear. They normally have a strong and distinctive smell and will stain housing and bedding materials. Examples are Jeyes Fluid, Izal, Stericol, Ibcol, Phisohex and Dettol.

Which disinfectant to choose?

There is a wide range of disinfectants available for use. When choosing a disinfectant to use, you need to consider:

- Can it be used for the species you work with?
- Which microorganisms does it destroy?
- Is it low risk in terms of health and safety?
- How quickly does it work?
- What dilution is it used at?
- How should it be stored?
- Will it corrode the housing?
- How easy is it to dispose of?

- What effects does it have on the environment?
- What does it smell like?
- How much does it cost?

Depending on where you want to use the disinfectant, the manufacturer may provide different dilution rates. There are often different dilution rates for general use and specific use.

Disinfectants for general use often work against a wide range of microorganisms and so are called **broad-spectrum** disinfectants. Disinfectants that are used specifically against a particular type of microorganism are called **narrow-spectrum** disinfectants.

What types of disinfectant are there?

Disinfectants are split into different groups according to the active compound that they contain:

- Phenols
- Aldehydes
- Peroxides
- Halogens

Phenols tend to be toxic to small animals and so are generally only used on farms and for large animal housing. Phenols may be black, white or clear, have a strong, distinctive smell and tend to stain housing and beds. Examples of phenols are Jeyes Fluid, Izal and Dettol. Phenol-based disinfectants should not be used for cats, rabbits or rodents.

Aldehydes work against a wide range of microorganisms and are highly toxic to living tissue. When making or disposing of them, you must take strict safety precautions as they can give off fumes. Examples include Formula H, Parvocide and Vetcide.

Peroxides are effective against a wide range of microorganisms. They are available as powders to be mixed with water for disinfecting housing and surfaces. Gloves and aprons should be worn when using this type of disinfectant. Once mixed, it is stable as a disinfectant for 5 days. Discard old solution and make up fresh as instructed. Examples include Virkon.

Halogens are effective if the instructions are followed correctly. They may irritate skin and so should be rinsed off thoroughly. Halogen disinfectants need to be made up frequently. Examples include bleach and other chlorine-releasing products, e.g. Halamid. Halogen-containing products are highly effective disinfectants if correctly used. Always follow dilution instructions for best effect as this chemical can be inactivated by incorrect dilution and by organic materials. They can cause irritation to tissues, so extreme care should be taken in preparation, use and disposal. Thoroughly rinse off any surface that has been in contact with this disinfectant. The product loses activity on exposure to air and light. New dilutions should be made up frequently.

Precautions to take when using a disinfectant include:

- Wear protective clothing and avoid contact with skin – gloves, apron and mask.
- Follow the safety instructions for using the disinfectant.
- Only use for the purpose recommended by the manufacturer.
- Use at the recommended concentration/dilution to achieve maximum effectiveness.
- Store the disinfectant in a secure location – preferably a lockable cupboard.
- Store the disinfectant in its original container with a tight-fitting lid to minimize the chance of leakage.
- Keep disinfectants away from children and animals.
- Wash hands thoroughly after use.

Manufacturer's instructions and COSHH sheets

It is vitally important to follow the manufacturer's recommended instructions as much research has been done on chemicals before they are released onto the commercial market in order to determine the safest use of the disinfectant.

All disinfectants should have an associated COSHH sheet that should be read prior to use and stored in a safe place in case of emergency. All staff should be made aware of any potential hazards that may be caused by the use of the disinfectant.

Dilution rates

Manufacturers always recommend dilution rates for the disinfectant. There may be more than one rate, depending on the usage and the microorganisms that need to be destroyed. Often, a routine strength is recommended with stronger rates for specific disinfections. Too weak a solution will usually be ineffective and too strong a solution is wasteful, and it may also endanger the safety of the patients.

Usually:

General cleaning strength = 1:100 (10 ml/l)
Broad-spectrum activity = 1:50 (20 ml/l)
Specific activity = 1:25 (40 ml/l)

Areas such as offices, corridors and reception areas should be cleaned using general strength. Areas such as theatres, waiting rooms, consulting rooms, runs and kennels should be cleaned using broad-spectrum strength.

How do disinfectants work?

Disinfectants for environmental use only destroy the micro-organism by disrupting its cell wall or contents in such a way that the microorganism will die or be killed by the chemical. The most resistant microorganisms are:

- Bacterial spores
- Some viruses (unenveloped)

The least resistant microbes are:

- Some viruses (enveloped)
- Bacteria (vegetative)
- Fungi

Disinfection and cleaning of the animal's environment

Animal housing and the surrounding environment can only be cleaned effectively if both physical and chemical action is taken.

Physical action (scrubbing) is most important for several reasons:

- Removes foreign materials such as blood which are ideal breeding grounds for pathogens.
- Disinfectants must have direct contact with the pathogen to be destroyed in order to be effective.
- Disinfectants are only effective once all other debris has been removed.

What is needed for cleaning animal housing?

- Dustpan and brushes
- Waste bags
- Scrubbing brushes
- Hot soapy water
- Buckets/hose pipe
- Clean water
- Disinfectant

To maximise the effect of the disinfectant being used and to prevent inactivation by organic materials, the following rules apply when disinfecting housing, surfaces and furniture within enclosures:

What is the correct way to clean animal housing?

- Remove animal to a safe place or pen them into a safe area.
- Remove all food and water containers and enrichment/toys.
- Remove soiled bedding/waste substrate into waste container (bag, wheel barrow or bin for example) and dispose of correctly.
- Soak all surfaces with hot soapy water.
- Scrub the soaked surfaces with scrubbing brush.
- Wash away all organic material and all soap with clean (preferably running) water.
- Apply disinfectant (made up at correct strength) and leave for the correct amount of time.
- Rinse off all disinfectant with lots of clean water if it needs to be.
- Leave to dry.

- Replace clean substrate/bedding.
- Replace all furniture for the enclosure after cleaning.
- Replace the animal safely and clean the holding pen/cage.

Antiseptics

Predominantly, antiseptics are used as cleansers for the skin and may also be called skin disinfectants. When applied to skin or mucous membranes of living tissues, antiseptics stop or prevent the growth of micro-organisms like bacteria and fungi but will not necessarily kill the microorganisms although some do.

Antiseptics are non-toxic to living tissue and are used prior to operations, before handling animals to prevent transfer of microorganisms and after handling contaminated material. They are also used to disinfect the patient's skin before and after surgery or after an injury where an open wound has resulted. Antiseptics work very quickly, and although they are not generally toxic, some can irritate the skin, and so it is important that they should only be used at their recommended dilution rate.

Which antiseptic to choose?

There are a range of antiseptics available for use, and choice will be affected by a number of factors in a similar way to disinfectants.

Types of antiseptic available

Quaternary ammonium compounds (QACs). There are two main types of QACs to choose from:

(1) Chlorhexidine plus a detergent property, e.g. Hibiscrub or Dinex
(2) Cetrimide, e.g. Cetavlon, Savlon or Vetasep

This type of antiseptic product is highly effective against microorganisms and has a rapid action as an antiseptic. They are often used as a preoperative skin cleaner and as a surgeon's scrub. They have a low toxicity to tissues but may be an irritant to some individuals. Recontamination by microorganisms is prevented for a time due to a residual effect. Use at recommended dilution and only on intact skin.

Iodophors – iodine-based compounds (e.g. Pevidine scrub, Betadine)

Iodophors are effective against skin microorganisms, non-irritant and have low toxicity to tissues. Their action is slow so length of time in contact with the skin surface is important. They can be inactivated by organic matter however. These types of antiseptic will usually stain the skin and any materials they come into contact with for a period of time following their use. Follow safety instructions for use.

Advantages and disadvantages of disinfectants and antiseptics

Disinfectants

Advantages	Disadvantages
More concentrated – increased efficacy Not so easily inactivated Broad spectrum of activity Added detergents to most	COSHH Can be toxic, e.g. phenols Can damage surfaces Expense versus economy May have long contact time

Antiseptics

Advantages	Disadvantages
Rapid action Tissue friendly Use on wounds and burns Safe for operator	Inactivated by organic material May irritate skin Can be contaminated and so grow bacteria

Alcohol gel

Alcohol hand gels are now routinely used in veterinary practices and other animal establishments as good practice in hand sterilisation prior to husbandry procedures occurring. Alcohol is a very effective agent against bacteria, viruses and fungi but has limited effects on the spores of these microorganisms. It is also effective against methicillin-resistant *Staphylococcus aureus* (MRSA) (see Chapter 21). Visitors to animal establishments such as zoos and farm parks are encouraged to use alcohol gels to sterilise their hands after handling animals or touching their enclosures. Alcohol can also be used as a surface cleanser in surgical areas of the veterinary practice. Care must be taken when using alcohol however as it is flammable and in excessive quantities can be an irritant. Repeated use can dry the skin, and so, those users that suffer from skin conditions such as eczema should take care in their use of alcohol gels.

Chapter 14
Basic Nutrition

Summary

In this chapter, the learning outcomes are:

- To identify the basic components of animal nutrition:
    - Proteins
    - Carbohydrates
    - Fats
    - Vitamins
    - Minerals
    - Water
- To identify considerations to be taken into account when feeding animals
- To identify how nutritional needs can be affected by life stages in animals
- To be able to describe nutritional differences between the dog and cat

Food or nutrients are required by the body in order to produce energy. Energy is necessary to drive the essential processes and systems in the body:

- Breathing
- Circulating the blood to tissues and cells
- Maintaining body temperature
- Muscle movement throughout the body
- The materials for repair, growth and reproduction
- General health

Nutrients are any food products that will support life. There are six major nutrient groups:

Animal Biology and Care, Third Edition. Sue Dallas and Emily Jewell.
© 2014 John Wiley & Sons, Ltd. Published 2014 by John Wiley & Sons, Ltd.
Companion Website: www.wiley.com/go/dallas/animal-biology-care

Those that can supply energy:

(1)   protein
(2)   carbohydrates
(3)   fats/lipids

Those which do not supply energy but are needed for its production:

(4)   vitamins
(5)   minerals
(6)   water

Animals eat in order to satisfy their energy needs. In the wild, when animals have eaten enough food to meet the body's energy demands, they will stop. However, due to the improved taste of pet foods, scraps from the human table and 'treats', some companion animals will eat in excess of their body's needs, resulting in obesity and other linked diseases. Many animals have a sedentary lifestyle with owners unable to provide sufficient exercise, which means that nutrients in excess of body needs will be converted to storage as body fat (*adipose tissue*).

Proteins

The sources of protein in an animal's diet can be of either animal or vegetable origin:

(a)   Animal origin
   - meat
   - fish
   - eggs
   - milk
(b)   Vegetable origin
   - soya and other pulses/beans
   - cereals

Proteins are large molecules, consisting of hundreds of single units called *amino acids* which join together to form chains. Dietary protein is broken down during the digestive process back into its amino acids. Proteins are made up of a combination of 23 amino acids. Animals need all 23 amino acids in order to maintain their body proteins. Some of these amino acids are obtained from the food they eat, and some are made within the body.

For example, dogs require ten amino acids to be supplied by the diet and can create or synthesize the remainder. Cats, however, require 11 amino acids to be supplied via the diet. The extra one (compared to dogs) cannot be synthesised by the cat and can only be obtained from animal protein. These dietary amino acids are referred to as *essential*.

Amino acids

- Arginine
- Histidine
- Isoleucine
- Leucine
- Lysine
- Methionine
- Phenylalanine
- Taurine (which the cat is unable to synthesise)
- Threonine
- Tryptophan
- Valine

Function of protein

- Energy (only used as an energy source if in excess or other energy sources are not available)
- Growth
- Repair of tissues
- Immune system to protect from disease
- Assisting metabolic reactions (enzyme and hormone)

Deficiency of protein in the diet

- Poor growth
- Weight loss
- Disease

Many tissues in the body rely on protein as a major component, e.g. hormones, enzymes, plasma proteins and antibodies. The quantities of protein required in the diet by an animal will vary according to:

- Species
- Age
- Sex
- Quality of the protein

The higher the biological value of a protein (in other words, the easier it is for the body to use), the smaller the quantity required. High-value protein includes:

- Egg
- White meat (chicken)
- Fish

After digestive disturbance or operations, it is usually recommended that high-value proteins are fed for a few days as they are easier to digest for the animal.

Low-value protein includes:

- Soya bean and other pulses
- Cereals

Excess protein in the diet cannot be stored but is converted by the liver to energy and nitrogenous waste (urea). This is then removed from the body by the kidneys.

Carbohydrates

The sources of carbohydrate in an animal's diet can be of either animal or vegetable origin:

(a) Animal origin
- milk
- milk powders
(b) Vegetable origin
- cereal starches (oats, lentils, rice)
- root vegetables (potatoes)

Carbohydrate can be divided into digestible (starches) and indigestible (dietary fibre or cellulose). Dietary fibre is found in plants and cereals and provides bulk to the faecal materials. It assists in regulating bowel function and the movement of undigested nutrients through the digestive tract.

Function of carbohydrates

- Energy
- Provides dietary fibre

Deficiency of carbohydrate in the diet

There are no related problems provided that other energy providing nutrients are available in the diet (i.e. fats or proteins). Carbohydrate is broken down in the digestive tract to simple sugars which are essential for most of the body's energy. If simple sugars are unavailable as a nutrient, the body can divert some amino acids to become an energy source. Simple sugars can be converted into a temporary stored form called *glycogen*. This is stored in the liver and muscles and converted back to simple sugar whenever its energy is needed by the body.

If the diet contains more carbohydrate than required for the production of energy, the surplus is converted into body fat and stored as adipose tissue.

Fats/lipids

The sources of fat in an animal's diet can be of either animal or vegetable origin:

(a) Animal origin
    - milk and other dairy produce
    - fish oil
    - fat of body origin (attached to meat)

(b) Vegetable origin
    - nuts
    - seed oils, i.e. sunflower, oil-seed rape and linseed
    - margarine

Function of fats/lipids

- Energy (a very concentrated form)
- Improved taste to the diet
- For the absorption, transport and storage of the fat-soluble vitamins – A, D, E and K
- Provide essential fatty acids (EFA) for body use

Deficiency of fat in the diet

- Reproduction problems
- Impaired wound healing
- Poor coat condition
- Dry skin

Fat is also called *lipid*. It is made up of glycerol, with attached fatty acids. Fatty acids are a very concentrated form of energy compared to protein or carbohydrates.

In the dog and cat, there are three EFA: linoleic, arachidonic and linolenic. Provided there is a dietary source, the dog can obtain or synthesise all three from any type of dietary fat. The cat, however, is only able to synthesise one EFA from the diet and must therefore be provided with a dietary source of the other two. Combined with the need to be supplied with one of the amino acids in the dietary food, this means the cat is considered a true carnivore. That is, it cannot maintain full health without a diet of animal tissues to utilise as a source of ready-made essential fatty or amino acids.

Body fat (adipose tissue) is created from a combination of fatty acids and simple sugars, if either is in excess in the diet.

Vitamins

Vitamins are important in the chemical reactions that go to make up metabolism. There are two groups:

(1) Fat-soluble vitamins – A, D, E and K (Table 14.1)
(2) Water-soluble vitamins – B complex group and vitamin C (Table 14.2)

Table 14.1   Fat-soluble vitamins.

Vitamin	Source	Function
A (retinol)	Fish oils, liver, egg and cereals	Night vision, body cell division
D (cholecalciferol)	Liver, fish oils, egg and cereals	Regulates calcium levels, bone growth and repair
E (tocopherol)	Vegetable oils, egg and cereals	Supports tissues and cells around the body
K	Developed in the intestines (no need for dietary source), green vegetables	Assists in blood clotting

Table 14.2   Water-soluble vitamins.

Vitamin	Source	Function
B1 (thiamine)	Cereals, organ meat, green vegetables, dairy products	Assists metabolic reactions, i.e. converts sugars to fatty tissues
B2 (riboflavin)	Organ meats, milk	Use and release of energy by cells
B6 (pyridoxine)	Cereals, meat and yeast	Metabolism of amino acids
B12 (cyanocobalamin)	Fish, organ meats	Blood cell production in bone marrow
Folic acid	Organ meats, fish; synthesised by gut	Blood cell production in bone marrow
Biotin	Produced by gut bacteria	Assists body metabolism
C (ascorbic acid)	Green vegetables; created in the body	Creates collagen for tissues, supports bone cells

Dogs and cats may synthesise most vitamin C required by the body, but primates, fish and guinea pigs are unable to do so and must receive a dietary source for body health and function.

Fat-soluble vitamins are stored in fatty tissues and in the liver and therefore could reach dangerous levels if given in excess. Water-soluble vitamins are not stored and must be supplied continuously via the diet and supplemented in medical conditions that lead to water loss, i.e. diarrhoea. Most species can produce vitamin C in the liver, but the guinea pig cannot and must be given vitamin C supplements routinely.

Minerals

The sources of mineral salts in an animal's diet can be of either animal or vegetable origin:

(a)   Animal origin
- dairy products
- meat

Table 14.3 Minerals.

Mineral	Food source	Function
Calcium	Milk, cheese, meat and bone	Nerve cell repair, muscle and bone formation
Sodium	Salt and cereals	Nerve and muscle activity, fluid balance in the body
Magnesium	Bone, cereals and greens	Bone formation and synthesis of protein
Phosphorus	Milk, meat and bones	Bone and teeth formation
Copper	Bones and meat	Red blood cell formation – haemoglobin
Iodine	Milk and fish	Formation of hormone from thyroid gland
Iron	Meat, eggs and greens	Red blood cell formation – haemoglobin
Selenium	Fishmeal, meat and cereals	Synthesis of vitamin E
Zinc	Meat and cereals	Tissue maintenance and aids digestion of food

- egg
- bone meal
(b) Vegetable origin
   - cereals
   - green vegetables
   - salt

Minerals are important for a variety of functions in the body. They are often referred to as *ash* on containers of pet food. Provided the animal is fed a balanced dietary product, minerals do not normally need to be supplemented (Table 14.3).

Minerals are divided into two groups:

(1) *Macro- or major minerals* (needed in large or regular amounts):
   (a) calcium
   (b) chloride
   (c) magnesium
   (d) phosphorus
   (e) potassium
   (f) sodium
(2) *Trace element minerals* (needed in only small amounts):
   (a) copper
   (b) iodine
   (c) iron
   (d) selenium
   (e) zinc

Function of minerals

- Assist in the maintenance of pH balance in the body
- Maintain the body's fluid balance

- Essential for the function of muscle tissues and conducting nerve impulses
- Help regulate the body's metabolism (via enzymes and hormones)

Never feed any one product in excess within an otherwise balanced diet.

Deficiency of minerals in the diet

Some minerals have an extremely complex relationship in the body, and if one is out of balance, it can affect the whole relationship. Deficiencies in minerals are often associated with excess minerals being added to the diet, i.e. calcium deficiencies can be caused by phosphorus excess in the diet. This could happen in animals being fed an excess of dietary meat or organ tissues.

If a good-quality diet (either commercial product or home recipe) is being fed, there should be no need to supplement vitamins and minerals to a normal healthy animal.

Water

Water is essential for all cells in the body and is found inside and outside all cells; 60–70% of an animal's body weight is water. It is involved with nearly every body process. As a result of the presence of water in the body, the following can take place:

- Transport of any material between tissues/cells
- Electrolyte balance
- pH balance
- Control of temperature
- Lubrication of all tissue cells
- A medium for blood and lymph

Water cannot be stored by the body and must be available all the time for all animals. Water in the body comes from:

- Food
- Drinking
- Chemical reactions (metabolism)

Water is lost from the body:

- In urine
- Via the lungs in breathing
- In faeces
- In sweat via the skin

It is important to stress that *fresh water must be available at all times for all animals.* This must be emphasised to all animal keepers. Some water will be available from canned food, but if a dry diet is given, the animal must receive water by drinking.

General considerations for feeding

- There are major differences in the dietary needs of each species of animal
- If the diet is balanced for that species, do not supplement vitamins or minerals
- The diet should provide enough energy for the animal, supplied by fats and carbo-hydrate rather than by diverting protein
- Energy levels and requirements will vary with age or life stages and activity levels
- Read instructions carefully before feeding dry diets in particular. Use a recommended 'measure' for quantities to prevent overfeeding

Figures 14.1 and 14.2 show a variety of food bowls available for the pet dog and cat.

Life stages for nutrition of the dog and cat

The main dietary components are:

- protein
- carbohydrate

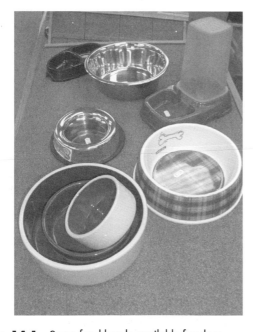

Fig. 14.1   Some food bowls available for dogs.

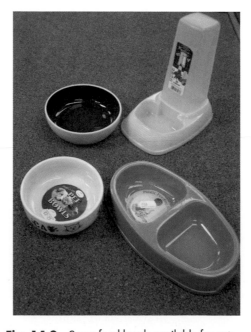

Fig. 14.2   Some food bowls available for cats.

- essential fats
- vitamins and minerals

These components provide energy following their breakdown in the gut and absorption. However, fat will provide twice as much energy as protein and carbohydrates. The quantities of the main components can be adjusted for any life stage in order to meet the demand of the animal (i.e. during growth phase, pregnancy and lactation) provided that the basic rules are understood.

Food provides energy but it is important that the nutrient content is balanced to the individual animal's requirements. The following stages need to be considered for the dog and cat:

- Growing puppies and kittens
- Adult maintenance
- Working dogs
- Senior dog and cat
- Pregnancy

Nutritional differences between the dog and the cat

Dog

Dogs are not true carnivores (meat eating); they have retained a number of molar teeth for chewing and grinding food which demonstrate this. Dogs can convert vegetable protein and fat into the ingredients necessary for body function. However, a vegetarian diet may not be balanced enough to maintain health in the long term. How the food supplied tastes, its energy content and its digestibility all need to be considered. A complete diet allows the animal to maintain body weight and fitness by supply of all the essential nutrients to meet whatever the daily needs of the animal may be.

Commercial proprietary diet types for dogs include:

- *Canned food* – meat and vegetable protein-based foods to be mixed with dog biscuits or meal for a complete diet
- *Complete semi-moist food* – similar to canned but can contain three times the calories of canned foods
- *Complete dry food* – have nearly all the water content removed, leaving them more concentrated than semi-moist foods and containing four times the calorie content of canned food. Some may need re-hydrating with water before being fed to the dog
- *Biscuits* – these are cereal based (providing carbohydrates) but also contain high levels of fat, vitamins, minerals and small quantities of protein
- *Treats* – are used for reward or snacks and are often very high in calories, colour and smell

Cat

The cat is unusual, having remained completely carnivorous (known as an obligate carnivore). As a result, protein will supply the majority of its energy requirements. This means that the dietary protein requirements for a cat are considerably higher than for a dog.

Commercial proprietary diet types for cats include:

- *Canned/foil-contained foods* – are meat or fish based, with some cereal (carbohydrates), fat, vitamins and minerals for a complete diet. The protein levels are much higher than in dog food.
- *Soft moist foods* – are supplied in pellet form containing meat, soya protein and some fats. These are usually packed in foil sachets.
- *Dry food* – resembles small biscuits containing fish and meat as a base, cereals, vitamins and minerals but tend to be low in fats. Fresh water must always be available for a cat fed on this form of diet.

All commercial proprietary diets and biscuit meal have full instructions for feeding, outlining quantities for all breeds and sizes.

Home-made diets

Home-made recipes for dogs and cats must still form a balanced diet. These can be time consuming to prepare. It is important to either mince or chop up food into small pieces for a cat diet because cats are unable to chew, they can only hold and tear food.

Examples of food sources in a home-made diet for a dog would include:
Proteins

- liver (high in phosphorus but low in calcium, rich in vitamins A and B)
- heart (high in fat, therefore used only in small quantities)
- chicken and turkey are lower in calories than other meats and easily digested
- fish is a good protein source but all bones must be removed (grill or steam but do not boil)
- egg (scrambled) is useful for recovery from illness and restoring appetite
- minced beef or lamb will include animal fat

Vegetables (seasoned, cooked carrot, cabbage and green beans) provide fibre, vitamins and minerals
Pasta, noodles and potato are good sources of carbohydrate but need flavouring

Feeding guidelines

(1)   Never feed bones of any kind
(2)   Feed a good-quality food product
(3)   Remove uneaten food daily
(4)   Always provide fresh water, changed daily
(5)   Check that the protein levels are correct for the animal's life stage and circumstance (to prevent upset to the gut and diarrhoea)
(6)   Serve food at room temperature for a dog and slightly warmed for a cat
(7)   Never feed raw egg white (a chemical in it makes biotin unavailable)

Table 14.4 Sources of nutrients.

Nutrient	Source
Protein	Muscle meat, milk, eggs, pulses
Fat	Animal fat, vegetable oils, some meats
Carbohydrate	Cereal, potato, pasta, rice

Nutritional balance

All foods supply energy. This is measured in units of heat (kJ/g or kcal/g). The foods of a dog or cat diet which provide protein, fat and carbohydrate (Table 14.4) all contribute energy. Protein and carbohydrate are equal in energy content, but fat will provide twice this amount of energy gram for gram weight.

The protein content of a diet must make up at least 20% of the total energy present in the diet in order for enough to be eaten for body maintenance needs.

Dogs and cats make use of fat in their diet. It is a rich source of energy and is required for the EFA needed for functions in the body. Fat is also stored as tissue around the body if fed in excess, to be used when food becomes short.

Carbohydrate is not required by the dog or cat but is used as a source of energy from cooked starches and sugars released from cereals, potatoes or pasta.

Dietary supplementation

Supplementation refers to foods that are provided as well as the normal ration and diet (Figs. 14.3 and 14.4). While some supplements may correct a deficiency in an animal with a medical disease, others may be used as:

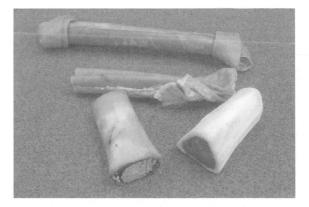

Fig. 14.3 Supplementary foods – chew types for dogs.

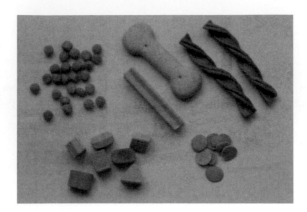

Fig. 14.4 Supplementary foods – biscuit types and shapes.

- Treats
- To increase food intake
- As a reward during training

Supplementation should not be used to improve a poor diet or be supplied in excess. A good-quality complete and balanced food will provide the nutrients required for health and fitness.

Growing puppies and kittens

After weaning, puppies and kittens need to be supplied, in their daily diet, with about 2–2½ times the nutrients required by an adult of the same breed/species. These increased requirements will gradually decrease as the animal becomes older and reaches adult weight.

Meals need to be frequent throughout the day (i.e. a 3-month-old puppy needs 4–6 meals), dividing the diet evenly between each one. The stomach size of young animals is too small to cope with only one or two meals a day. By 6 months of age, the frequency of meals is usually at 2–3 meals a day, down to 1–2 meals daily by 1 year of age for a dog. Cats tend to snack as adults and will often stay on 2–3 meals daily.

The previous information will vary from animal to animal. Owners generally notice that one of the meals for puppies and kittens is often not eaten; the food in that meal should then be spread through the remaining feeding times until the adult routine is reached.

When adult, usually, a pet dog will be fed once or twice daily, and a cat will be fed 2–3 meals daily, as required. A lot will depend on the type of food (canned, moist or dry) as to the feeding times, or an unlimited feeding method can be used in cats on dry diets.

Commercial foods are available in formulas for growing puppy and kitten needs. It is important that food chunks are appropriate in size to the animal. Texture is also important: with only milk (or deciduous) teeth, a large amount of chewing is not possible.

Adult

Once established, feeding routines should not be altered in timing, place or diet types. To do so is stressful to an animal and appetite may decrease as a result. Feeding times should never be too late in the evening, because the animal may need to urinate or defaecate within 3–4 hours of eating, by which time it may be shut in and the owners in bed.

Commercial diets all have information on feeding and quantities, but if part of the ration is always left uneaten, reduce the amount of food until all is eaten at each meal. To maintain the animal's interest, many owners supplement the diet with meal scrapes, gravy, etc. Cat foods are produced in many flavours, some owners using a different one for each day of the week. The condition, energy levels, health status and body weight of the animal need to be monitored to ensure that the diet suits the individual animal. If any change in the diet is considered, always introduce the new diet slowly over a number of days, overlapping it with the old diet to avoid any gut upset.

Working dogs

Depending on the training, working, resting times and function, working dogs may need quite different diets and feeding routines.

A working dog that runs long distances each day may need as much as two to three times the normal recommended adult ration of food, e.g. sheep dogs that may run more than 20 miles a day.

Generally, diets are grouped for carbohydrate or fat requirement. Carbohydrates (i.e. cereals as biscuits) release sugars and are useful for dogs that require energy for short duration, i.e. agility dogs, both in practice and competition.

Other working breeds that are active for long periods and in all weather conditions will need more energy for running and to hold the body temperature in extreme cold (sheep dogs and sledge dogs). Fat increase in the diet is ideal for these dogs. Protein in increased amounts may be useful for muscle development, but the energy requirements will come from carbohydrate and fat. Diets that have increased carbohydrate and fat levels are often referred to as 'active diets'.

Working dogs are normally fed only a small meal before work, leaving the main meal of two-thirds of the required daily intake to be fed after a rest period, allowing time for proper digestion.

Senior dogs and cats

Older animals will vary in condition and health status considerably. There are many commercial diets on the market to choose from. Depending on the health of the animal, some are for use with specific medical diseases; others are more generally restrictive of some nutrients for cases of obesity. These obesity diets are often referred to as 'light diets or reducing diets'.

Older animals may have sight, taste and smell losses, as well as poor appetite, poor teeth and gum condition, all making eating difficult. Many also have reduced movement of food in the gut, leading to constipation problems.

To provide for the nutritional needs of these senior animals, consider:

- Improving the taste/smell of the food by warming it to body temperature
- Using one of the appropriate senior diets on the market (seek veterinary advice first)
- Increased fibre in the diet to prevent constipation, i.e. use of bran
- Use of easily digested high-quality proteins, such as fish, poultry and egg, in the diet base
- Encouraging the animal to eat the daily ration by hand feeding initially
- Feeding small meals throughout the day (up to six), in order for the animal to eat the whole daily ration

For any animal, it is important to care for the teeth to encourage eating by preventing the build-up of tartar on the teeth, also check for loss of, or loose, teeth, gum disease and inflammation. All these will affect the animal's ability to eat. Many dogs and cats will allow the owner to clean their teeth with a soft toothbrush or finger brush, but if this is not possible, a teeth de-scale and/or teeth removal by a veterinary surgeon may be required.

Mobility problems and joint disease, in dogs particularly, may make bending to the food and water bowls difficult or impossible. To assist the animal, raise the food and water bowls off the floor on to a low box (Fig. 14.5) with a ridge around the edge (to prevent the bowls falling off). These can be home-made or bought from most pet shops (Fig. 14.6).

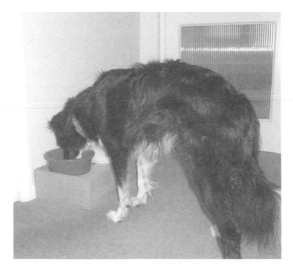

Fig. 14.5 Food bowls on a low box.

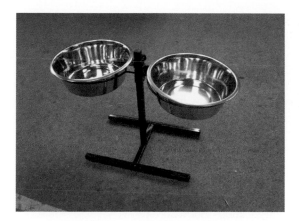

Fig. 14.6   Raised bowl system that can be bought from pet shops.

Pregnancy

Dogs

For most of the pregnancy, it is not necessary to increase the quantity of food, provided a balanced, good-quality food product is being used.

It is only during the final 3 weeks of pregnancy that an increase in food intake is required. This is at the time of most weight gain and growth occurring in the foetuses. Overfeeding before this stage of pregnancy may lead to fat deposits; weight gain as a result may lead to problems during parturition (birthing/whelping):

- Increase food by 10–15% per week from 6 weeks of pregnancy until parturition. This increases total food intake to approximately 50% over maintenance levels of food being fed
- Use diets formulated for pregnancy and lactation needs
- Feed small meals and often in the final 2 weeks of pregnancy, to assist food intake
- Provide fresh drinking water, at all times

Cats

From the time of mating, diet quantities need to be increased for the pregnant cat to approximately 30% above maintenance amounts. Cats will rarely overeat; therefore, food can be constantly available as requirements increase:

- Feed a diet formulated for a cat during pregnancy and lactation or alternatively add kitten food to the diet as this contains the higher level of protein required by the mother
- Ensure food is always available (referred to as free-choice feeding); this will help the cat to eat sufficient nutrients
- Provide fresh drinking water, at all times

How much should be fed?

The amount to be fed is based on energy needs and the rate of conversion of food to energy (metabolism) by the individual animal.

Take the number of kcal (kilocalories) of energy needed by an animal and refer to the content tables on any pre-packed food. The manufacturer will use the kcal/day requirements to suggest the amount in weight (grams) of the diet to feed with regard to the percentage value of nutrients in that food.

As a general guide for dogs:

- Small: 250–750 kcal/day
- Medium: 1000–2000 kcal/day
- Large: 2000–2500 kcal/day

Chapter 15
Handling

Summary

In this chapter, the learning outcomes are:

- To be able to identify reasons for handling animals
- To identify the importance of the correct approach when handling animals
- To be able to describe suitable examples of animal handling and restraint procedures for a range of species

Domestic species of animal will usually need handling at some point during their life. It is necessary to appreciate the behavioural differences between species in order to perform handling safely. Body language is quite complex in some species, i.e. the dog, and must be taken into account before approaching the animal.

Handling may give rise to fear and stress in the animal, which could be due to a learnt response following a bad handling experience. Any knowledge of the individual's temperament or behaviour in given situations and previous required handling is helpful information.

Possible reasons for handling

- Daily, weekly, monthly checks etc.
- Grooming
- Transportation
- First aid situations
- Examination after injury
- Medicating

Animals should be accustomed to handling from an early age. Teaching the animal to tolerate having difficult areas, such as ears, feet and mouth, looked at will make life less stressful for animal and handler at a later date.

Animal Biology and Care, Third Edition. Sue Dallas and Emily Jewell.
© 2014 John Wiley & Sons, Ltd. Published 2014 by John Wiley & Sons, Ltd.
Companion Website: www.wiley.com/go/dallas/animal-biology-care

Approaching an animal for handling

- Assess the animal's behaviour and body language.
- Be quiet but confident to establish control of the situation.
- Talk in a reassuring manner.
- Never corner the animal; always leave supposed choices.
- With a dog or cat, reach out to introduce yourself to the animal with a loosely clenched fist, palm facing the floor.
- Stroke the animal and accustom it to voice and scent but be aware that some animals may be head shy.
- Only lift the animal if the approach has been accepted.
- Handle with minimum restraint, especially cats.
- If the animal becomes or is aggressive, then a firm method of restraint is needed for the safety of handlers.

Examples of behaviour seen when animals are unwilling to be handled

- Cats – hiss, adopt defensive posture, growl, strike with front claws and flatten their ears to the skull and dilation of the pupils.
- Dogs – hackles raised, growling, lips in snarl position, ears forward, barking and attempting to bite.
- Rabbits – biting, scratching using hind legs, thumping hind legs on floor and, if terrified, squealing.
- Guinea pigs – are not aggressive but will stampede or circle their housing in an effort to get away.
- Small rodents, e.g. rats, hamsters and gerbils – bite if startled or hurt.

Handling procedures

It must be remembered that there are different handling techniques available and these may be used within the animal industry. The information given in the following text are examples of effective, safe, suitable methods that do not compromise the welfare of the animal being handled and also ensure safety of the handler.

Rat

Place hand firmly over the back and rib cage and restrain head with the thumb and forefinger immediately behind the lower jaw (Figs. 15.1 and 15.2).

Guinea pig

Grasp under the trunk with one hand while supporting the hindquarters with the other hand (Fig. 15.3). Bring towards you and rest on your chest in order to promote security for the animal – keep one hand over the shoulders and one hand under the hindquarters.

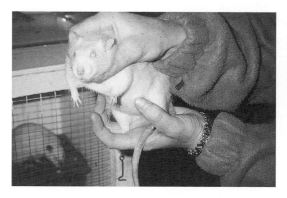

Fig. 15.1 Correct holding technique for a rat.

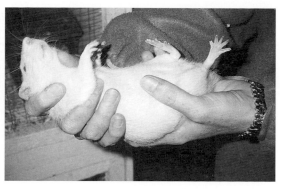

Fig. 15.2 Correct holding technique to expose the abdomen and chest.

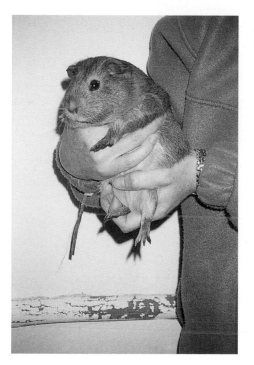

Fig. 15.3 Holding technique for a guinea pig.

Gerbil

Never lift by the middle or end of the tail. The tail is firmly grasped at the base and the gerbil is lifted and cradled in the palm of the hand. Use the over-the-back grip to prevent struggling (Figs. 15.4 and 15.5). Alternatively, if the gerbil is used to being handled, use an over-the-shoulder grip to pick the gerbil up.

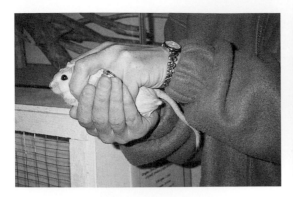

Fig. 15.4 Holding a gerbil.

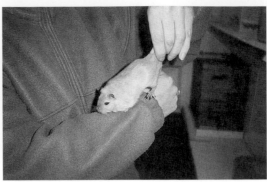

Fig. 15.5 Restraint for a gerbil.

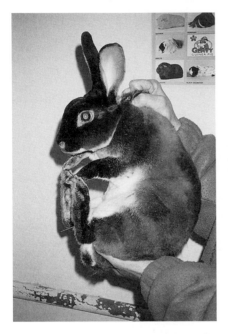

Fig. 15.6 Correct lifting technique for rabbits.

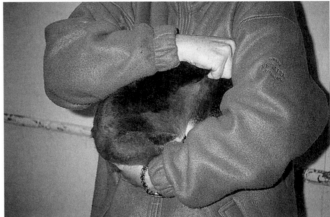

Fig. 15.7 Correct technique for moving a rabbit longer distances.

Rabbit

Never ever lift a rabbit using only the ears:

- *Short distances* (for cleaning housing) – grasp the skin over the neck with one hand and support the hindquarters with the other (Fig. 15.6).
- *Longer distances* – having lifted the rabbit from housing using the previously described method, it is positioned against the handler with its head tucked under the handler's arm, the hindquarters being supported by the handler's arms (Fig. 15.7).

An alternative method that can be used in both situations described earlier is put one hand on the shoulder of the animal and slide your hand over and underneath so that the first finger is positioned between the front legs of the rabbit. The thumb and middle finger can then close over the forelegs of the rabbit, and the handler's other hand can be used to lift the hindquarters. The rabbit can then be lifted and either placed in a carrier, on a handling table for examination or cradled against the handler's chest or along their arm. Never lift a rabbit to the point where it can try an escape over the shoulder of the handler; otherwise, severe scratching can occur to the handler and the rabbit risks injuring itself.

Dog

Before handling, always check the following:

- The collar is correctly fitted and will not slip off.
- Position of additional restraint device if required, e.g. Halti® or other head collars, cage muzzle, nylon muzzle or harnesses (correct size/correct fit).
- Temperament (muzzle if necessary).
- Reason for handling.

To apply a tape muzzle to a dog:

- Two handlers are required, one to hold the dog and one to apply the muzzle.
  - o Dog handler
    - ■ Stands facing the same way as the dog and to one side (alongside the shoulder).
    - ■ Takes hold of the scruff and collar (if worn) with both hands, behind the dog's ears.
  - o Person applying tape muzzle
    - ■ Use a bandage which will not stretch.
    - ■ Cut a length in excess to requirements.
    - ■ Make a loop with a double throw knot (Fig. 15.8).

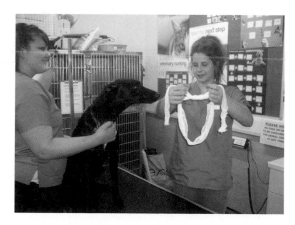

Fig. 15.8 Make a loop with the tape muzzle, with a double throw knot.

- To tape muzzle a dog.
- Keeping the loop open, approach from the side of the dog.
- Drop the loop over the dog's mouth and nose and tighten the loop quickly (Figs. 15.9 and 15.10).
- Cross the muzzle ties under the jaw.
- Knot the ends behind the dog's ears and tie into a bow for quick release (Fig. 15.11a–c).

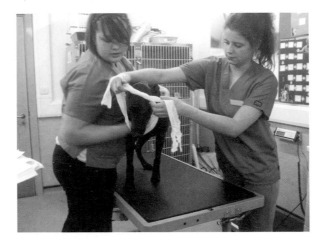

Fig. 15.9 Drop the loop over the dog's mouth and nose.

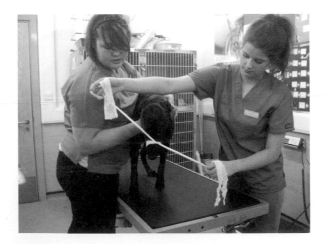

Fig. 15.10 Tighten the loop over the muzzle.

(a)

(b)

(c)

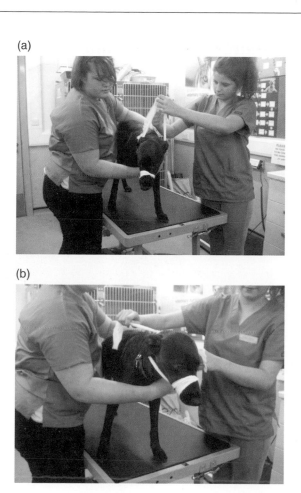

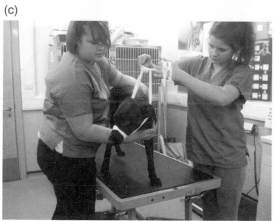

Fig. 15.11   (a–c) Knot the ends behind the ears and tie a bow for quick release.

Restraint procedures in the dog and cat

For intravenous injection

- Presenting one of the forelegs for procedures such as an injection into the vein or taking a blood sample (Figs. 15.12a, b and 15.13).

For subcutaneous injection

- Using the scruff area on the back of the neck (Figs. 15.14 and 15.15).

(a)   (b)

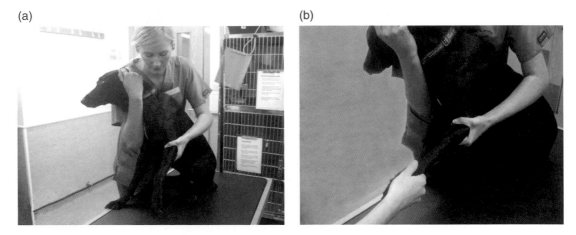

Fig. 15.12   (a) Position for i.v. restraint. (b) Place thumb over the upper part of the leg and rotate the vein from medial to cranial surface.

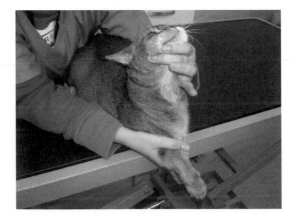

Fig. 15.13   Restraint by one person of a cat for i.v.

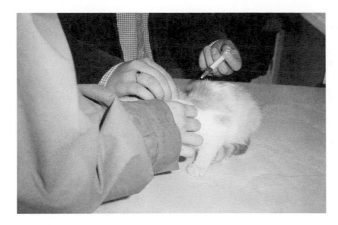

Fig. 15.14   Cat in sitting position.

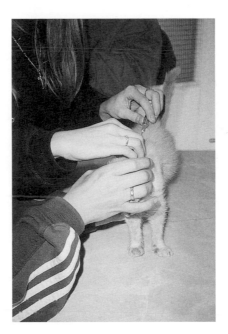

Fig. 15.15   Cat in standing position.

For intramuscular injection

- Using the muscle on the front of the hind leg. Never use the muscle at the back (caudal aspect) of the hind leg, to prevent damage to the main nerve supply (sciatic nerve). Two handlers are required, one to control the head and one to give the injection (Fig. 15.16).

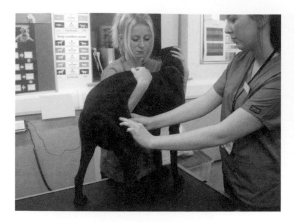

Fig. 15.16 Dog standing – restraint for injection into the front/cranial part of the upper hindlimb.

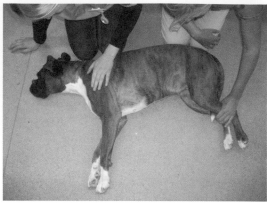

Fig. 15.17 Restraint for access to the limbs, chest or abdomen.

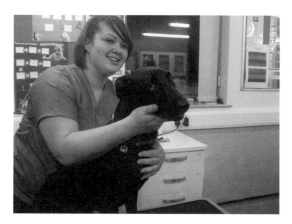

Fig. 15.18 Controlling the head standing to the side.

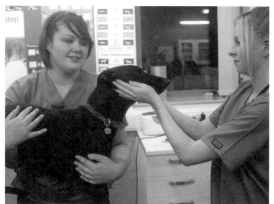

Fig. 15.19 Controlling the head standing in front.

On its side (lateral position)

- To expose the limbs, chest or abdomen (Fig. 15.17).

For general examinations

In these situations, the head must be controlled (Figs. 15.18 and 15.19).

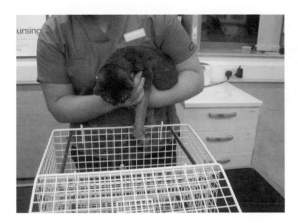

Fig. 15.20 Lifting cat from carrying cage.

Approaching a cat

- Use calm, confident movements.
- Speak quietly all the time.
- Attempt to stroke the head first and then along the cat's back.
- When the cat responds (non-aggressively), pick the cat up by placing one hand under the cat's chest and the other hand under the cat's hindquarters (Fig. 15.20).

Transferring a cat from basket to examination table or surface

- Place one hand under the chest and, supporting the hindquarters, lift.
- Hold under one arm, hand still under the chest, and transfer other hand to support and control the cat's head.
- Alternatively, this hand could scruff the neck to control the head.
- Never over-restrain a cat unless really necessary.

Chapter 16
Grooming and Coat Care

Summary

In this chapter, the learning outcomes are:

- To identify the reasons for an animal to be groomed
- To identify the aims of grooming an animal
- To describe the factors affecting coat growth
- To identify and describe the coat types in dogs and cats
- To name and describe the use of a range of grooming equipment
- To describe a grooming procedure including bathing and drying

One of the many responsibilities of a dog or cat owner is that of coat care. As breeds of dog and cat were developed for size, character and colour, so their coat length, texture and density evolved. Careful management of these many and varied coat types is part of the owner/pet interaction. Often, the choice of breed is based on a dog or cat seen in a breed book, but it is essential to investigate the amount of time and frequency of coat care required. There is a vast difference in the time it takes to groom a Doberman and an Old English Sheepdog and a Siamese and a Persian cat.

Reasons for grooming

- Show
- Hygiene
- Work
- Welfare
- Acceptance in society

Animal Biology and Care, Third Edition. Sue Dallas and Emily Jewell.
© 2014 John Wiley & Sons, Ltd. Published 2014 by John Wiley & Sons, Ltd.
Companion Website: www.wiley.com/go/dallas/animal-biology-care

Main aims of grooming

There are a number of aims when grooming an animal:

- To remove dead hair
- To clean the coat and skin
- To remove knots, mats and tangles

Grooming dogs

Grooming covers the following factors:

- To encourage bonding and trust between an animal and its handler
- To improve the handling of the animal
- To monitor the general health of an animal
- Allows opportunity for identifying health problems such as external parasites (fleas/mites) and skin problems (lumps, bumps, etc.)
- To monitor the condition of the nails

The dog's coat

The earliest breeds of dog evolved in the northern hemisphere and so needed a dense coat for protection from the cold. As dogs moved further south to the warmer climates of the world, their coat became thinner and shorter to allow the dog to function in extreme heat. Selective breeding further enhanced coat features for specific breeds and purposes. Table 16.1 shows different coat types.

Every breed varies in the type of coat hair it has. Hairs grow in hair follicles with several hairs to each follicle. Usually, there is an outer coat composed of *primary* or *guard hairs* and an undercoat made up of secondary hairs. Often, the undercoat is finer than the outer coat. Hair will be shed periodically. The growth rate of hair varies from breed to breed.

Other factors which influence the growth of hair are as follows:

Seasons

- *Spring* – triggers production of the summer coat, causing the old winter coat to be shed. The coat is oily, due to an increase in the sebaceous gland activity in the skin.
- *Autumn* – triggers the production of the much denser winter coat, causing the summer coat to be shed. The coat is less oily due to reduced sebaceous gland activity.

Environmental temperature

- Dogs kept in centrally heated housing will shed their coat continuously. Dogs kept in outside kennels will shed in spring and autumn.

Table 16.1 Examples of coat type in the dog.

Type	Hair length	Breeds	Grooming frequency
Smooth (Fig. 16.1)	Short and fine	Chihuahua	Minimal grooming
		Boxer	Twice weekly
		Doberman	Weekly
		Whippet	Weekly
		Pointer	Weekly
	Long and dense	Labrador	Twice weekly
		Corgi	Weekly
Double (Fig. 16.2)	Medium to long	Collie	Daily and weekly
		German Shepherd	Daily and weekly
		Old English Sheepdog	Daily and weekly
Wiry (Fig. 16.3)	Short	Dachshund	Weekly
		West Highland White	Weekly
	Long	Airedale	Daily and weekly
		Schnauzer	Daily and weekly
Silky (Fig. 16.4)	Short	Spaniel	Daily and weekly
		Pekinese	Daily and weekly
	Long	Afghan	Daily and weekly
		Yorkshire	Daily and weekly
Woolly/curly (Fig. 16.5)		Bedlington	Daily and weekly
		Poodle	Daily and weekly
		Kerry Blue	Daily and weekly

Daily indicates the coat should be briefly groomed once a day.
Weekly means the coat should be thoroughly groomed once a week.

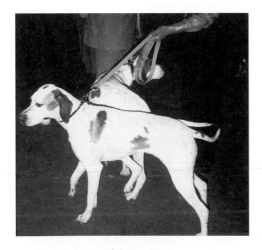

Fig. 16.1 Smooth coat – Pointer.

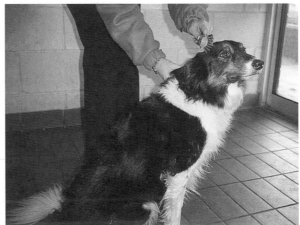

Fig. 16.2 Double coat – Collie.

Ill health

- If the animal becomes debilitated due to acute or chronic illness, the coat growth cycle will be interrupted.

Diet

- A balanced diet with all essential nutrients will ensure normal coat growth and condition.

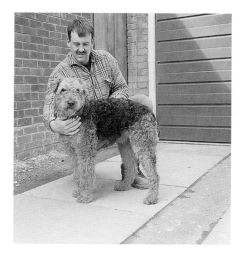

Fig. 16.3 Wire coat – Airedale.

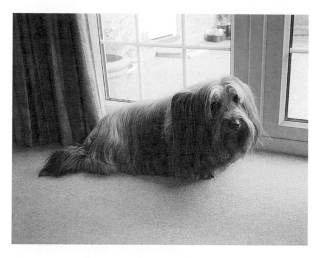

Fig. 16.4 Silky coat – Skye Terrier.

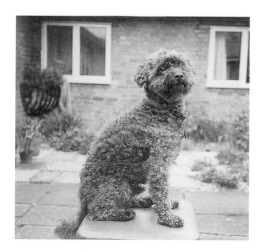

Fig. 16.5 Woolly/curly coat – Poodle.

Hormone levels

- Levels will alter during oestrus in the bitch, slowing the rate of growth. The coat texture can alter in some disease conditions which affect the body's hormone levels, not only causing the coat to grow more slowly but also making it coarse and rough to touch.

Grooming for different coat types

There are a number of different coat types in dogs. The coat type depends on the proportion of different hair types within the coat. Knowing the coat type of the dog is important as it allows the right products to be selected during the grooming process.

Smooth coat

A true smooth coat is smooth and sleek in appearance with minimal undercoat. The smooth coat type can be short as in the example of a Whippet or long as in the example of a Labrador. Matting of this type of coat does not occur due to its short length. However, the coat will become clogged with dead hair when moulting. Increased grooming at this time will keep the skin in good condition. To prevent loss of natural oils in the coat, only bath if really necessary. If the coat is muddy, brush it out once the coat is dry.

Equipment required:

- *Short coat* – use a hound glove
- *Long coat* – use a comb and a bristle brush

Double coat

In a double coat, the topcoat and undercoat are of equal length. The coat tends to stand off the skin to create a fluffy appearance. Very often, the coat is quite waterproof. This coat type will matt and tangle if not groomed frequently. Regular grooming sessions of up to three-quarters of an hour to one hour may be necessary to prevent the coat tangling.

Some breeds in this category, for example, the Old English Sheepdog, are clipped to about 2.5 cm in length in order to simplify grooming. This summer clip will allow the dog to cope better in hot weather.

Bath as a maximum three to four times yearly (the preference is twice yearly), in spring and autumn to condition the coat and clean the skin. Brush out mud once dry and regularly comb out the undercoat during the moulting season.

Equipment required:

- Bristle brush
- Slicker/carder brush
- Comb

Wiry coat

A true wiry coat feels harsh to the touch. The coat is dense in nature. To avoid matting of the coat, these breeds need regularly combing. To keep the coat wiry, the topcoat should be hand stripped and plucked two to three times per year. Alternatively, it may be machine clipped at 3 monthly intervals, followed by a bath to condition and clean the skin. It should be noted that clipping will make this type of coat become softer to the touch. Should mats occur in a wiry coat, work them out carefully with the correct dematting equipment. As a wiry coat grows, if it is not hand stripped in time, it gets softer and is said to have blown.

Equipment required:

- Slicker/carder brush
- Comb
- Dematting comb

Silky coat

A silky coat is usually medium long in length and soft and fine to the touch. Without frequent attention, these coats become very tangled. The coat is so fine in these breeds that it is hard to untangle even with dematting combs. Spaniels and Afghan hounds must have the dead coat hair stripped out every 3–4 months. At this time, the coat is usually trimmed, paying particular attention to ears and feet. The fine hair in the ear canals should be plucked at regular intervals and the foot hair trimmed to reduce mud and the attachment of barbed grass seeds.

Bath as required to help both grooming and skin condition, using an appropriate shampoo.

Equipment required:

- Bristle brush
- Dematting comb
- Slicker brush

Woolly/curly coat

Woolly/curly coat is often referred to as a non-shedding coat. The coat tends to be dense and profusely curly. The coat doesn't moult but grows continuously. As the hair grows, it becomes trapped, and so, regular grooming is a must for this coat type. These breeds need clipping and bathing every 6–8 weeks. If not groomed out, the dead hair will form a feltlike mass. The ear canals need regular plucking to prevent mats which soon plug with earwax and may lead to infection if not attended to.

Equipment required:

- Comb
- Slicker/carder brush
- Dematting comb
- Scissors

Grooming equipment

Every dog needs its own grooming equipment, normally bought when setting up a new puppy. Equipment to choose from includes the following:

- Brushes:
  - (a) Bristle brush
  - (b) Slicker/carder brush
  - (c) Hound glove
  - (d) Rubber brush
- Combs:
  - (a) Fine comb
  - (b) Wide-toothed comb
  - (c) Rake comb
  - (d) Flea/louse comb
  - (e) Dematting comb

- Cutting equipment:
  - (a)   Stripping knife or comb
  - (b)   Thinning scissors
  - (c)   Scissors
  - (d)   Electrical clippers
  - (e)   Nail clippers

Brushes

Bristle brushes are available in a range of sizes and shapes. The handle is made of either wood or rigid plastic, with synthetic or natural bristles. The bristles are set close together, making this an ideal surface-only brush. It is unable to penetrate dense coats but is ideal for smooth coats and the removal of mud or other surface material stuck to the hair. On short smooth coats, it can be used with pressure on areas of the dog's back, flanks and hindquarters. The main effect of this surface brushing is to stimulate the skin and distribute the natural oils from the skin to the hair shaft ends, giving a shine to the coat.

Pin brushes are available in a range of sizes. The handle is made of either wood or a rigid plastic. The pins, often with plastic-coated tips to prevent scratching the skin surface, are set in a flexible rubber-backed cushion. The pin brush will separate hairs and lay the coat in position, particularly useful for the silky long coats and double coats. These brushes also stimulate the skin, distributing the natural oils from the skin to the tips of the hairs. If the coat has tangled hair or knots, then use a comb first to remove these before brushing. This will prevent the coat being pulled or broken when the pin brush is used.

Slicker/carder brushes (Fig. 16.6), with a wooden or rigid plastic handle, come in a range of sizes. The pins are hooked and set in a rubber-backed cushion, giving some flexibility to the grooming movement. The function of these hooked pins is to remove dead coat. No pressure should be applied when using the slicker brush because the pins could easily scratch or damage the skin surface. It can be used on a range of coat types from silky to double and in some body areas of curly and wire-coated breeds. Never use on areas of the body where the coat is normally thin such as the stomach, groin or armpits.

A *hound glove* (Fig. 16.7) fits over the groomer's hand like a mitten or glove, as the name suggests. It is made of flexible plastic or rubber with short bristles made from wire or plastic, and some have a velvet-type surface on one side and bristles on the other. It is used to remove dead or moulting hair (bristle side) and to polish the coat (velvet side) in smooth and short-coated breeds. Care should be taken when using the bristle side, in case too much pressure is used and the skin is damaged.

Combs

Combs are used to remove dead hair and prevent mats forming behind the ears, in the neck/collar area and over the hindquarters.

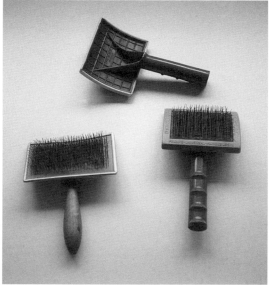

Fig. 16.6 Slicker/carder brushes.

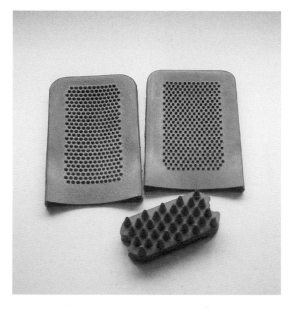

Fig. 16.7 Hound glove (top) and rubber brush (below).

Combs are available made from metal or plastic, with or without handles (Fig. 16.8), with solid teeth or rotating teeth. Some combs are half wide toothed and half fine toothed so that each half can be used in different body areas and on different coat types. The teeth tips are rounded or plastic coated to avoid tearing the skin surface. Some combs also have pins set so that they are able to roll individually and prevent coat damage when in contact with a mat or tangle.

Combs should be used carefully, especially when encountering a knot or tangle. Slowly tease the hairs and never rush this stage or the coat will be pulled, hurting the dog and making it unwilling to be groomed.

Rake combs (Fig. 16.9) have ridged metal teeth with round tips, set perpendicular to the handle, and resemble a small garden rake. They should not be used by pressing into the coat. Their function is to break up mats and, in dense coats, lift and remove dead undercoat hair. They are pulled towards the groomer through the coat and in the direction of the coat hair.

Flea combs have fine teeth set close together, with a grip area. These are pulled slowly and carefully through the coat, going with the normal coat direction. If a parasite is encountered, the gap between the teeth is too small for it to pass through so it is lifted onto the comb for the groomer to remove.

Dematting combs (Fig. 16.10) have wooden handles and teeth which on one side are rounded and blunt and on the other side are a series of cutting blades. These combs are used, with extreme care, to cut through large mats of hair by placing the blunt side against the dog's skin surface and with a gentle sawing action cutting away from the skin surface and through the mat. This will allow the matted areas to either be combed out or further subdivided for combing and removal of the dead hair.

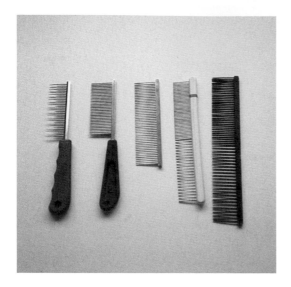

Fig. 16.8 Comb types.

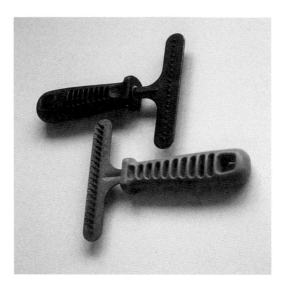

Fig. 16.9 Rake comb.

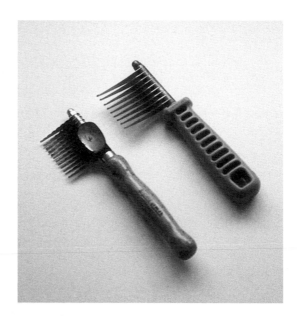

Fig. 16.10 Dematting comb.

Cutting equipment

A *stripping knife or comb* (Fig. 16.11) is used to remove dead hair and at the same time trim the live hair. The comb has a serrated metal cutting edge, set against a guard plate on one side for the removal of dead hair. The stripping knife has a metal handle and blade. Sections of coat hair are held between the operator's thumb and the blade, and

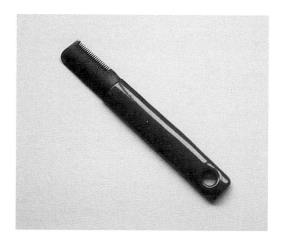

Fig. 16.11 Stripping knife.

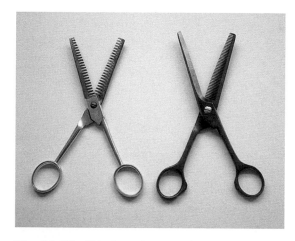

Fig. 16.12 Thinning scissors or shears.

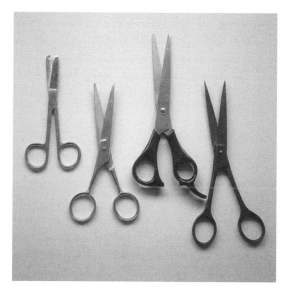

Fig. 16.13 Scissor types.

the blade is pulled away from the skin with a twisting movement. At the same time, dead hair can be pulled or plucked. This is known as hand stripping and is used on wire-coated breeds such as terriers, Wire-haired Dachshunds and Schnauzers. If done correctly, it is not at all painful.

Thinning scissors (Fig. 16.12) have one regular and one serrated blade or both blades serrated. They thin the coat without affecting its appearance. These scissors are therefore used on the undercoat, preserving the colour of the outer coat appearance.

Scissors (Fig. 16.13) are available in many sizes and shapes for use on the various body areas, from long, sharp, tapering blades to short, blunt-ended blades, depending on

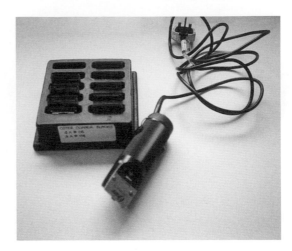

Fig. 16.14 Electrical clipper with range of blades.

the area that requires a trim. Blunt-ended scissors are used to trim between toes and in delicate areas around the eyes, ears, lips and genitals.

Electrical clippers (Fig. 16.14) are used by professional groomers in conjunction with scissors, particularly in the curly-coated breeds such as the Poodle. These coats keep growing all year round and need constant attention. Always keep the blade of the clippers flat to the coat to avoid cutting the skin. The clipper cuts away the excess hair more rapidly than scissors and is used with a variety of detachable blades. The blades vary from fine tooth for close trims to ones set with wide-spaced blades or teeth, which leave short hairs against the skin surface. The blades are snapped onto a post on the clipper only when the clipper is running. The clipper is held like a pencil which gives a firm grip, allowing the groomer to move over the coat lightly and keep the blade flat against the section being clipped.

Clippers will get hot during use so it is important to closely monitor the blade temperature in order to prevent a clipper burn or rash developing on the damaged skin surface. There are several ways of avoiding this:

- Spray hot blades with aerosol lubricant spray to reduce temperature.
- Change the hot blade for a new cool blade.
- Use a second clipper, allowing the first to cool.
- Keep the blades in use sharpened.
- Only clip hair that is completely dry.

Nail clippers (Fig. 16.15) are only used to cut nails which are overlong. A range of clippers is available, from the guillotine clipper (also useful in small mammals) to the double blade type. The choice of nail clipper will depend on the length and position of the nail presented.

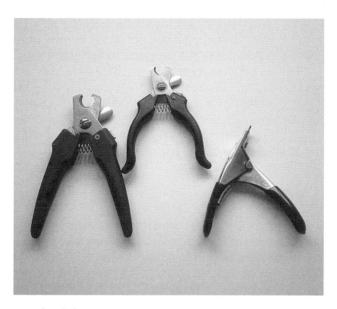

Fig. 16.15 Types of nail clippers.

Grooming procedure

Depending on the coat type of a dog, grooming will be a daily and/or a weekly event. It provides the owner with the opportunity not only to condition the coat and skin but to:

- Clean any discharge and examine the eyes
- Check and clean the ear to prevent infection developing
- Clean and examine the mouth and particularly the teeth
- Examine and trim any overlong toe nails
- Check the anal region

The *eyes* should be bright and free of any discharge. If any discharge is seen in the corner of the eye, moisten a clean piece of cotton wool with water and wipe away in the direction of the nose. If the discharge looks anything other than clear, check for signs of inflammation and seek veterinary attention.

The *ears* should be free of wax, a dull pink colour and without odour. In the curly-coated breeds, the ears need to be plucked free of hair which, if left in place, attracts wax, parasites and infection. Check for signs of discomfort or reluctance by the dog when the flap is being examined, which may indicate a problem.

For the *mouth*, the gums and tongue should be pink (pigmented in the Chow Chow) or partly pink with pigmented areas. The gums should be well defined around each tooth, with no food or other materials attached. In order to prevent any build-up of tartar on the teeth, pet toothpaste in various flavours and toothbrushes can be used as part of the daily grooming examination.

The *feet* or paws should be clean around the nail bed, nails just in contact with the ground, and excess hair cut short between the pads and nails to prevent mats and grass seed barbs penetrating the skin and causing an abscess.

The *anal region* under the tail and around the anus needs to be checked daily in dogs, whether short or long coated. The area should be free of any faecal material and show no signs of redness or inflammation. Should the dog start licking excessively around the anal region or scooting on its rear end, the anal glands should be checked for a blockage. These glands are situated on either side of the anus and may not empty as expected when the dog defaecates, leading to infection.

Nail clipping

Active healthy dogs do not need frequent nail clips. The nails will wear naturally with everyday use on paved surfaces. The exception may be the dewclaw, which can grow round into the nail bed if left unchecked, although they tend to be slow growing in most breeds.

The nails may need attention if:

- The dog is exercised only on soft ground or grass
- The dog is elderly
- Due to limb injury, the dog walks with uneven gait
- A nail becomes broken or damaged

Nail clipping is a process that many people are scared to do, but once you have learnt, then it is quite straightforward. Care must be taken not to cut the "quick" in the nail. The quick is the blood vessel running down the centre of the nail. If this blood vessel is caught, then bleeding can be stopped quite quickly. It is better to cut a small amount at a time if you are unsure. Once an animal has had a bad experience during nail clipping, then it can react badly on future occasions.

Equipment needed

- A pair of nail clippers
  - o There are a range of styles on the market from small scissor type nail clippers to plier type and guillotine type. There are also electric nail grinders that can be used. Use the type that you feel most comfortable with.
- A coagulant powder should be available.
  - o A coagulant powder helps to stop bleeding if clipping causes the nail to bleed. There are a number of brands commercially available e.g. Quick Stop, Styptic Powder, Trimmex
- A nail file
  - o Nail files can be used at the time of clipping to smooth off any rough edges. They can also be used on claws in between trimming sessions to smooth any breaks or flaked nail edges. Nail files can be used to trim the sharp ends of claws, particularly dew claws.

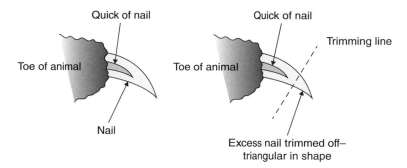

Fig. 16.16 Nail trimming guide.

Nail clipping process

- Choose the right type of clipper for the job – one that you feel comfortable with – pliers type or guillotine types are commonly used.
- The size of clipper used will relate to the size of claw being cut. If you use clippers that are too big for the claw, then you can damage the claw. If the clippers are too small then you will not get a full cut through the nail which can be painful for the animal.
- Restrain the animal appropriately and reassure throughout by staying calm, being confident and talking in a calm manner to the animal.
- Locate the 'quick' in the animal's claw. This can be easily seen if the claws of the animal are white but it is trickier in animals with dark claws. If the animal has dark claws, it is necessary to examine the shape of the claw and identify a cutting position approximately 0.5–1 cm in front of the quick. A rule of thumb is to identify a triangular shape at the end of the claw (Fig. 16.16).
- Holding the claw firmly at the base to prevent any twisting, quickly cut the claw using firm pressure in order to minimize any trauma for the animal. Avoid cutting the 'quick'. Always ensure you can see where the blades of the claw clippers are to avoid cutting too much off at once.
- If the quick is cut apply a coagulant powder such as quick stop to the bleeding claw. If no powder is available, apply firm pressure to the end of the claw until bleeding stops.
- Check the nail afterwards for sharp edges and if any are present, then use a nail file to gently smooth the sharp edges.

Brushing the coat

Once the general checks are complete, brushing and combing in preparation for the bath can begin. It is essential to brush and comb before the bath to remove all matted and tangled hair. Shampoo and drying make matting much worse in some coat types. Check through the coat with a wide-toothed comb to ensure no tangles are left.

Start the procedure with:

- The hind legs
- Then the forelegs

- Back to the tail section and tail
- The body coat, one side at a time
- Chest area
- Lastly the head, face and ears

When brushing, pay particular attention to the groin area and the armpit area on the forelegs where mats may develop. The head and ears in breeds such as Poodles, Spaniels, Lhasa Apso and Afghan need particular attention. The ear hair is long and fine and tends to form small mats.

The eye area on breeds such as Pekinese and Shih Tzu needs particular attention and care as these are short-nosed breeds (*brachycephalic*) with protruding eyes. As a last resort, it may be necessary to remove mats and tangles with scissors or electrical clippers, especially if it is clearly painful to the dog or the dog is becoming aggressive due to the grooming.

Bathing

Reasons for bathing:

- To control skin parasites
- To clean soiled coat
- To remove odours
- To improve coat appearance for showing
- As part of a medical treatment
- To mask the scent of oestrus

Equipment needed for bathing includes:

- Cotton wool to plug ears (optional)
- Shampoo/conditioner
- Mixer hose or jug
- Bath with non-slip mat
- Towel or dryer

Ear plugs – After brushing and combing, ear plugs may be placed in the ear canal to prevent the entry of shampoo and water. This is optional and should not be used if upsetting to the dog.

Shampoo – There is a wide range of shampoo on the market available for different coat types, different coloured coats, etc. If in doubt, use a general-purpose shampoo unless the coat requires otherwise. Conditioners may be used to improve the coat texture and make it more manageable for final brushing when dry.

Shampoos available include the following:

- *Mild* – have only low levels of detergent to avoid eye or skin irritation.
- *Medicated* – prescribed by a veterinary surgeon in cases where the dog has skin problems. These shampoos contain antiseptics such as iodine to reduce skin bacteria levels or drugs to assist a specific skin condition.

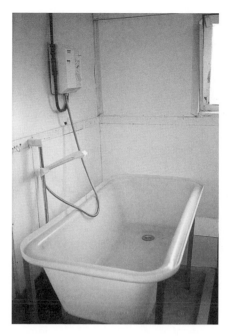

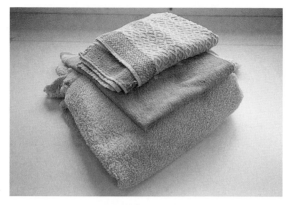

Fig. 16.18 Have several towels available.

Fig. 16.17 Dog bath with shower hose.

- *Insecticidal* – for control of surface/skin parasites such as lice, fleas and ticks. These are often used in combination with parasite control programmes that use spot-on, tablet or injection methods.
- *Colour enhancing* – used to improve the appearance of coats, particularly white ones.
- *Conditioners* – used to prevent tangles in long-haired coats and improve the brushing-out process once dry. Used in show dogs such as Yorkshire Terriers, Maltese Terriers, Afghans and Shih Tzus.

Always decant the shampoo required into a plastic container (such as an old washing-up liquid bottle) as this allows easy application of the shampoo, used either concentrated or diluted. If the shampoo should be knocked and fall, there is no risk of broken glass, and the noise of the container falling will not frighten the dog.

Mixer hose or jug – The use of a hose with a shower head allows the water pressure and temperature to be regulated (Fig. 16.17). If a hose is not available for rinsing, then use a jug.

Bath – A household bath can be used, with a hair catcher over the plughole to prevent blockage, or a child's paddling pool. Always provide a non-slip surface to prevent the dog from damaging the bath surface if it slips or panics. Rubber bath mats or car mats can be used.

Towels or dryer – Several towels are needed for any breed other than small or toy (Fig. 16.18). Always provide more than required to avoid having to leave a half-dry dog to shake off the excess water over all surfaces. In winter, place the dog in a warm area to dry once excess water has been removed from the coat using towels. Household hand-held hair dryers (Fig. 16.19) may be used but be careful introducing the dog to the dryer as the noise and warm airflow may frighten it. Never hold dryers too close or use a high-temperature high-flow setting:

- *Floor dryers* – mounted on stands and are powerful, quickly drying heavy-coated breeds (Figs. 16.20 and 16.21).
- *Cage dryers* – attach to the front of holding kennels and cages. These are used after towel drying.
- *Wall-mounted dryers* – similar to the hand-held dryer but more powerful and space saving. A hose applies the 'blow dry' effect when directed on to the dog's coat.
- *Cabinet dryers* (Fig. 16.22) – box cages with a false, vented floor, containing the blow dryer. Warm air flows, fan assisted, into the box area where the dog sits.

Bathing technique

Make sure before bathing starts that all the equipment required is to hand. Never encourage a dog to jump into or out of a bath in case of injury – always lift the dog safely into the bath, ensuring the correct lifting technique is used. Do not leave an animal unattended in the bath in case the animal panics.

Use a collar restraint to attach the dog to the bath, leaving both the groomer's hands free. A nylon collar and lead should be used, never a chain. If the dog panics or slips, the nylon lead can be cut quickly, preventing injury.

The groomer should wear protective clothing and non-slip soles to shoes or boots, for safety. When using medicated and parasite shampoo, gloves should be worn by the groomer to protect their skin:

(1) Place a non-slip mat into the bath area.
(2) Lift the dog into the bath. Two people may be required to lift medium and large breeds.
(3) Regulate water flow and temperature.
(4) Soak hindquarters first, using the hands to force water through heavy coats.
(5) Continue soaking, moving last to the head and face, protecting the eyes and ears from the water.
(6) Once the dog is soaked, introduce the shampoo, using hand and sponge. As before, start over the hindquarters and move towards the head, including the abdomen, under the tail and between the foot pads but still protecting the eyes at all times.
(7) Hold the head up to encourage water and shampoo to drain back along the spine while attending to the face and chin.
(8) Rinse off the shampoo.
(9) Repeat the application of shampoo (if medicated or parasite shampoo, leave in contact with the skin for correct amount of time).

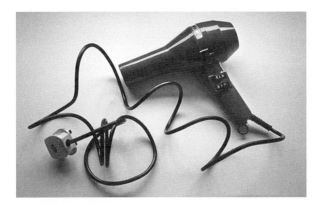

Fig. 16.19 Hand-held dryer.

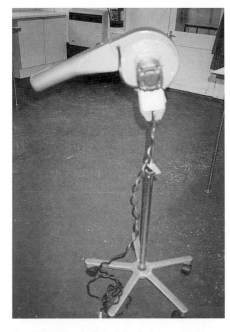

Fig. 16.20 Type of floor dryer stand.

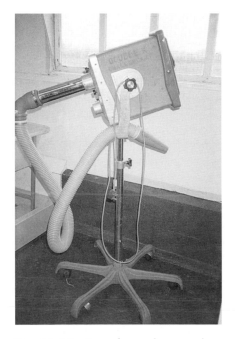

Fig. 16.21 Type of cage dryer stand.

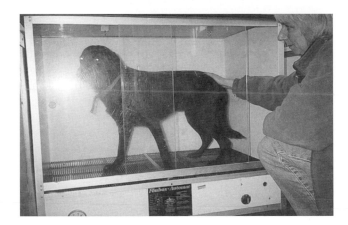

Fig. 16.22 Cabinet dryer with false vented floor.

(10) Rinse thoroughly from head to toe.
(11) Squeeze water out of coat using hands or chamois-type cloth.
(12) Towel dry on a non-slip surface and place in a warm area to finish drying or dry using a dryer.
(13) Pat dry, and never rub vigorously with long coats as this will create tangles.

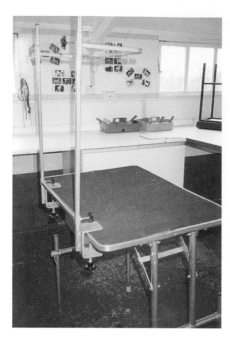

Fig. 16.23 Grooming table.

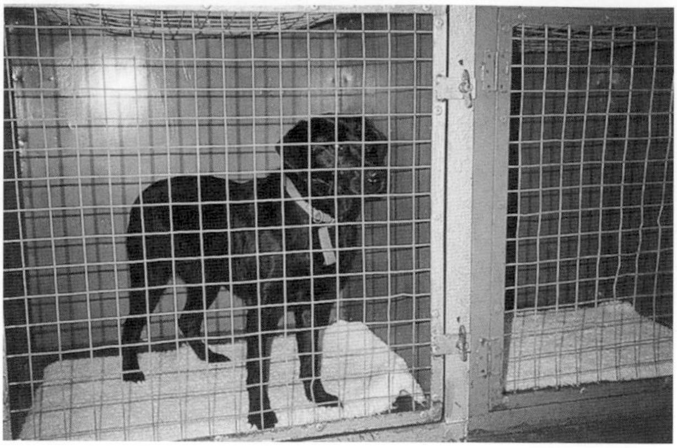

Fig. 16.24 In the holding kennel awaiting collection by owner.

During the drying stage, the coat can be brushed out. The objective of using the dryer to dry some breeds is to get the coat as fluffy as possible. To achieve this, the coat is dried in sections, brushing constantly to straighten curls.

Finally, trim nails if necessary and clip hair between foot pads. Professional groomers would then proceed with the plucking, stripping, clipping and scissoring required by certain breeds, depending on coat type and requirements. This would be done on a grooming table (Fig. 16.23). The dog would then be transferred to the holding kennel to await collection by the owner (Fig. 16.24).

Cats

Grooming provides the owner with the opportunity not only to condition the coat and skin but to:

- Clean any discharge and examine the eyes
- Clean the ears and check for signs of infection, excess wax or ear mites
- Examine the mouth and check the teeth for build-up of tartar and for gum disease
- Examine and trim claws and clean claw bed of caked-on dirt
- Clean dirty coat
- Check for skin parasites

Grooming should begin from the time of weaning to accustom a kitten to short but daily coat care. As with the dog, this also becomes a bonding/playtime session between the owner and the animal. This attention is particularly important if the kitten is to be a show animal.

Cats spend a considerable part of every day in self-grooming. They have a specially adapted tongue with backward-facing barbs for the removal of dead hairs from the coat.

Grooming in cats will:

- Remove dead hair
- Remove material from coat surface
- Stimulate skin and distribute secreted oils for coat condition
- Provide a feeling of well-being

Constant grooming in long-haired cats can cause health problems. During self-grooming, the cat will swallow large quantities of saliva and wet hair, which forms *hair balls* or sausage-shaped plugs in the stomach. This ingested hair can cause an obstruction in the digestive tract. In the event of loss of appetite, weight loss or constipation, contact a veterinary surgeon for advice.

The cat's coat

Selective breeding and genetic mutation have enhanced cats' coats or caused coat loss. The cat has a topcoat of *guard hair* and an undercoat which consists of coarse, bristly *awn* hairs and soft downy hairs.

Examples of coat types in cats are as follows:

- *Short hair*, e.g. British short hair, has short guard hairs with even shorter but slightly curly awn hairs as a sparse undercoat.
- *Long hair*, e.g. Persian, has extremely long guard hairs with a thick undercoat of downy hair which gives this breed its full, dense coat.
- *Semi-long hair*, e.g. Ragdoll – similar to a long-haired coat but mid-length. Possesses a thick undercoat of downy hair which thickens the coat during the colder months.
- *Curly coat*, e.g. Cornish Rex, has very short curly awn and downy hairs of the same length and no guard hairs at all.
- *Wire hair*, e.g. American Wirehair, has short curly, even coiled guard hairs, down and awn.
- *Hairless*, e.g. Sphinx, which has a coat so sparse as to appear hairless but in fact has a covering of downy hairs on the legs, tail and face only.

The cat has three kinds of skin gland to care for its coat. Two types are sweat-producing glands, some located only on the pads of the feet and others over the entire body used to leave its scent and mark territory. Territory marking is seen when the cat rubs against objects. The third type of gland is the sebaceous gland near the hair follicles which secretes sebum to help waterproof the coat.

Moulting occurs in the spring and autumn, when the coat comes out in what seem like handfuls at a time. Long-haired coats will moult all year round due to the constant room temperatures in which these cats tend to live. It is therefore essential that the long-coated breeds have owners who realize the necessity of daily grooming routines.

Grooming in cats

Short coat

These cats are efficient self-groomers, with the normal-shaped head giving a slightly longer tongue than in the long-coated breeds. Two half-hour grooming sessions per week are ideal. In between, continue to condition the coat by stroking along the lie of the hair or polishing the coat using a piece of silk, velvet or chamois leather cloth.

Equipment required:

- Fine-toothed comb
- Soft bristle brush
- Rubber brush (see Fig. 16.7)
- Chamois cloth

Long-haired and semi-long-haired coat

These cats tend to have shorter faces resulting in shorter tongues, therefore making these breeds tend less efficient self-groomers. Moulting all year round, the coat tends to mat. Grooming is needed daily, split into two half-hour sessions during the day to check for mats. Start with a normal comb to remove dead hair and then use a fine comb to fluff up the coat. A toothbrush is used to brush the face hair, keeping well clear of the eyes.

Equipment required:

- Wide-toothed and fine-toothed combs
- Slicker brush
- Bristle brush
- Toothbrush – medium bristle

Curly coat

Curly coats should not be overgroomed as this could result in baldness. A soft brush with short bristles is sufficient for removal of dead coat. Groom twice weekly.

Equipment required:

- Soft bristle brush

Wire coat

These cats have a crimped, woolly coat which is coarse to the touch. Removal of the dead hair in a wiry coat is essential but ensure that the curls spring untangled back into position. This is achieved by minimum brushing with a soft bristle brush and hand stroking at least twice weekly.
Equipment required:

- Soft bristle brush

Hairless coat

With hair only on the extremities, skin conditioning is more essential in these breeds. Do not brush these breeds. The skin needs daily sponging to remove *dander* (small scales from the hair and dried skin secretions). A sponge moistened with warm water wiped over the body daily or more frequently if required will remove the dander which, if left, could cause a skin allergy.
Equipment required:

- Sponge

Bathing a cat

Groom out all mats and hair contaminated with faeces. If these mats cannot be groomed out, it may be necessary to cut them off with scissors.

As with a dog, make sure all equipment is to hand before starting. A non-slip surface in the bath is essential in order to give the cat something to cling to. Unless bathing is a routine experience, cats can find it very traumatic so only bath them if really necessary.

Two people are required, one to hold and reassure and one to bath:

- Fill the bath with about 10 cm of warm water into which the cat is lowered gently.
- A mixer hose and/or a sponge are used to soak the coat hair and apply the shampoo. Proceed with a thorough rinse and then wrap the cat in a towel.
- At all times, make sure water or shampoo never gets close to the eyes, ears or mouth.
- Wipe over the face with cotton wool moistened in warm water.
- Towel dry and keep in a warm area until fully dry.
- If the cat will tolerate it, use an electrical dryer set only to warm and held at a safe distance.
- Once the coat is dry, comb out gently and brush.

- Finish with the grooming of the coat hair.
- *Short hair* – start at the head and comb/brush towards the tail, including chest and abdomen. Then, rub down with a chamois or nylon pad to polish the coat.
- *Long hair* – comb the legs free of tangles; then the abdomen, flanks, back, chest and neck; and then the tail section, fluffing out the coat hair by brushing the wrong way. Finally, using a toothbrush, groom the face hair.

When all grooming is complete, remove the dead hair from the combs and brushes, wash, disinfect and rinse before storing to prevent cross infection between grooming sessions or infecting another animal groomed with the same equipment.

Equipment should be sterilized on a regular basis also.

Warning

If the coat is dirtied by chemicals such as tar, creosote, paint or oil, remove as soon as possible to prevent absorption through the skin or self-grooming and ingestion of the chemical, which may be a poison. Never use chemicals to remove these substances. On a dry coat, use soft margarine, washing-up liquid or liquid paraffin to work the substance free of the hairs, then proceed with a bath and dry thoroughly. If the cat has self-groomed, contact a veterinary surgeon immediately for advice.

Chapter 17
Other Animals Kept as Pets

Summary

In this chapter, the learning outcomes are:

- To identify and describe basic husbandry considerations for a range of animals kept as pets including:
  - Small mammals
  - Birds
  - Fish
  - Reptiles, amphibians and invertebrates

Across the UK, cats and dogs make up the major proportion of pets kept in UK households; however, small mammals, birds and fish are also kept in large numbers. Over the last decade, keeping reptiles, amphibians and invertebrates as a hobby has also increased substantially. If working in the animal industry, it is likely that, at some point, all these animals will be encountered within a collection, and so having knowledge of their care and husbandry is important. Beyond pet ownership, the care of some of these species can be very intricate, and it may be necessary to take expert advice in some cases, e.g. fish.

Basic husbandry for other animals

Housing

There are a range of housing options (cages, runs, tanks, pens, vivaria, aquaria) for small mammals, birds, fish and reptiles available in the current market (2013). Choice *should* be made according to suitability for the species and practicalities of hygiene, but there is often an aesthetic appeal for the owner/carer/keeper that is part of the final decision made.

Animal Biology and Care, Third Edition. Sue Dallas and Emily Jewell.
© 2014 John Wiley & Sons, Ltd. Published 2014 by John Wiley & Sons, Ltd.
Companion Website: www.wiley.com/go/dallas/animal-biology-care

Whatever housing option is chosen, it must be safe and secure for the animal. The following aspects for the housing should be considered:

- Constructed soundly of materials suitable for the species being housed:
  - ○ No sharp edges
  - ○ No rough surfaces
  - ○ No loose joints
- Easy to clean
- Easy to provide food and water
- Comfortable for the animal intending to be housed
- Enrichment is able to be placed within the housing in order to mentally stimulate the animal
- Escape proof for the animal intending to be housed
- Prevents other animals from getting in
- Large enough for free movement of the animal and allows a moderate amount of exercise, e.g. a rabbit in a hutch should be able to stand up on its back legs and have space between its ears and the roof of the housing. A bird should be able to sit on a perch in the cage and have head clearance and tail feather clearance and also be able to stretch its wings up and out without them touching the sides of the cage
- Dry and well ventilated
- Methods for heating or cooling as required during seasonal changes in environmental conditions, without being subjected to extremes of temperatures, e.g. direct sunlight entering the housing – this is particularly important in the case of reptiles that are not capable of maintaining their own body temperature and so are reliant on external heat sources
- Lighting requirements can be met
- The animal can excrete away from the bedding/food areas
- Suitable drainage

Promoting health

- Regularly examine the animal to determine health status or detect injury. If any animal is found to be diseased, it is important to move it to isolation or quarantine areas
- Only purchase animals from reputable and reliable sources in order to avoid disease being brought into the existing animal establishment
- Clean housing thoroughly and disinfect regularly
- Move any sick animal to isolation
- Apply high levels of hygiene to all equipment used in the housing
- Have a good airflow through the housing to prevent breathing problems and air-borne diseases
- House different species separately where possible
- Change bedding several times a week, depending on species

Nutrition

The needs of each species of animal have been well documented. However, there are general guidelines:

- Feed only fresh and clean foods
- Check that the feed container is in date, has not been broken open or damaged and is not contaminated by anything
- Feed must provide all the nutrients necessary for full health
- Water is fresh and always available
- Water containers/feeders are cleaned regularly
- Food is stored in closed containers at room temperature and kept dry

Small mammals

Small mammals that may be kept as pets include rabbits, guinea pigs, hamsters, gerbils, rats and mice.

Handling of these species must be done with care to avoid injury to the animal and the handler. If these types of animal are not used to regular handling, then they may bite or scratch, and so a basic knowledge of handling for each species is important to ensure the welfare of the animal. Initial restraint of these species should be firm but gentle to prevent injury (Fig. 17.1).

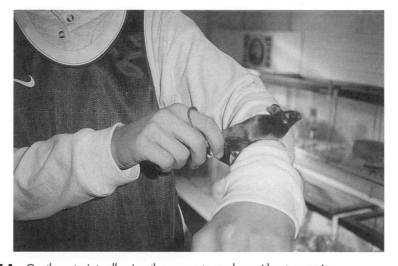

Fig. 17.1   Gentle restraint, allowing the mouse to explore without escaping.

Rabbits

Rabbits (*Oryctolagus cuniculus*) belong to the order Lagomorpha, and since their domestication, there have been many different characteristics selected for. Rabbits are popular pets and there are over 80 breeds to choose from, with variation in shape, colour, size and character. Rabbits can usually fall into three main categories:

- *Normal* – these breeds have a coat type of short, dense fur, similar to that of the wild rabbit, and were bred originally for meat, e.g. New Zealand White, Chinchilla, Dutch (Fig. 17.2) and Californian
- *Fancy* – mainly bred for show, with distinguishing features, e.g. Lop for their large ears, Netherland Dwarf and Flemish Giant for their size and Himalayan for their coat markings
- *Rex and Satin* – noted for their velvet- or Satin-like coats in which the guard hairs are missing or below the under-hair level, giving the coat a smooth, dense appearance

Rabbits are social animals if reared with their littermates and should not be kept on their own if possible. In the wild, they live in groups with a well-defined hierarchy. The males will fight to defend territory if kept in the same housing, as they would in the wild. Females will live together happily, but are likely to show dominant aggression once maturity is reached. Most owners pair up male and female, with one or both neutered if not intending to breed from them. Sometimes, rabbits can be paired with other species, such as guinea pigs, but this is not always ideal because the rabbits do tend to bully the guinea pig (being a smaller animal); also, the two species have different nutritional requirements, making feeding difficult. A rabbit kept alone needs a lot of human interaction to prevent fear or aggressive behaviour. To enable this, some single rabbits are trained to use litter trays and are kept as house pets.

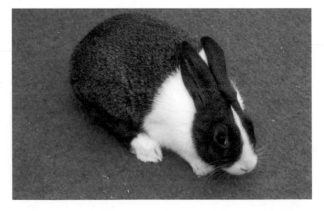

Fig. 17.2 Dutch rabbit (short coated).

Biological data: Rabbit

Male	Buck
Female	Doe
Offspring	Kits (kittens)
Adult weight	1–10 kg (depending on breed)
Maturity	12 weeks onwards
Gestation period	28–32 days
Litter size	2–7 (average size)
Weaning age	6 weeks
Body temperature	38.5°C
Life span	6–8 years (average)

Anatomical facts: Rabbits

Eyes

- Rabbits have a wide field of vision, 190° for each eye. Dilation of the pupil means their night vision is about seven to eight times more effective than that of humans.

Ears

- Have a good blood supply and assist with body heat regulation and sound gathering.

Teeth

- Dental formula: incisors 2/1, canines 0/0 (diastema or gap), premolars 3/2 and molars 3/3.
- Rabbit's teeth are open rooted, continuing to grow throughout their life. If the correct foods and environment are provided, the teeth are continually worn down, which is essential for health. Rabbits are classified as herbivores; this effectively means that their diet consists mostly of plant matter. Therefore, the diet must be high in fibre.

The teeth are adapted to bite, chew and grind the high-fibre diet. It is because of constant wear and tear that the teeth continue to grow during the animal's life.

The upper incisors are chisel shaped and grow roughly at a rate of 2 mm/week. The two pairs of upper incisors (Fig. 17.3) are situated one behind the other. The upper hind incisors are called peg teeth. They are intended to be worn away by the lower incisors; in a normal, healthy rabbit, this effect gives the teeth their sharp chisel edge.

Body cavities

- The thoracic cavity is small, allowing for a large abdomen, which houses a lengthy intestinal tract with a large caecum.

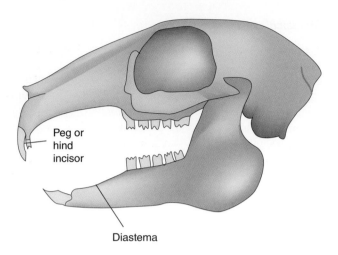

Peg or
hind
incisor

Diastema

Fig. 17.3 Rabbit skull: detail of mouth.

- The digestive system of a rabbit has evolved to ensure that maximum benefit is derived from their diet. Digested foods pass through the stomach, into the small intestines and onto the caecum. This is a sac-like structure near the junction of the small and large intestines. It contains active bacteria that break down plant fibre (cellulose) for digestion and absorption. Many nutrients would be lost to the body at this point; however, the rabbit overcomes this loss by passing these nutrients in the form of soft caecal pellets (produced at late night/early morning) from the anus and eating them directly from the anus (referred to as *coprophagia*). The swallowed caecal pellets are mucous covered and stick together to pass through the digestive tract, allowing further breakdown and absorption of any useful nutrients. The rabbit then passes the characteristic dry, hard faecal pellet. This process of passing nutrients twice through the digestive system allows for maximum extraction of nutrient material.

Skeleton

- Light, delicate bones are covered with a powerful muscle system, especially to the hind legs. This can mean that the limbs and spine are prone to fracture, if handled carelessly. Rabbits can also cause substantial injury with their hind legs due to the power transferred through the limb.

Scent glands

- Located in the anal region for marking of territory.

Handling rabbits

If handled regularly, correctly and gently, a rabbit will become tame quite quickly.

- Rabbits are easily frightened and must be handled carefully and securely.
- If a rabbit feels insecure or is handled badly, it will struggle violently potentially, causing serious injury to both the handler and itself.
- Rabbits should **never** be picked up by their ears as this will cause them pain and distress and potential severe injury.
- Nervous rabbits should be scruffed gently with one hand, while the other hand lifts the rump. Once lifted, nervous rabbits can be supported along the forearm of the handler with their head tucked against the body under the elbow until the rabbit can be placed on a non-slip surface (Fig. 17.4).
- Tame rabbits can be lifted by putting one hand under the chest and holding the forelegs separately between the thumb and the two fingers while supporting the rump with the other hand. Once lifted, support the rabbit by holding against your chest before placing onto a non-slip table. Keep control of the rabbit on the table by placing your hands around its body.
- Rabbits must not be allowed to struggle violently as they may break their backs by kicking and twisting.
- It is advisable to replace a rabbit in its housing backwards to avoid a last kick back as it is released.

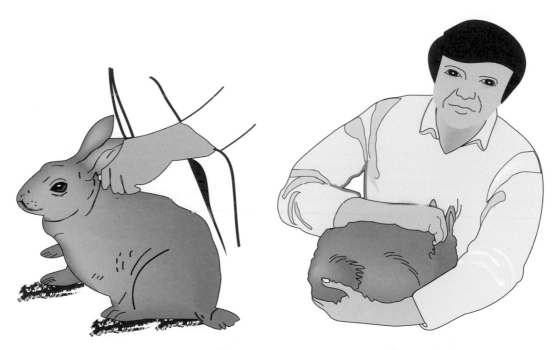

Fig. 17.4 Methods of handling and restraining a rabbit. Source: Adapted from Ferris, M. (2003) Pet Store Management Course Manual. Reproduced with permission of The Pet Charity.

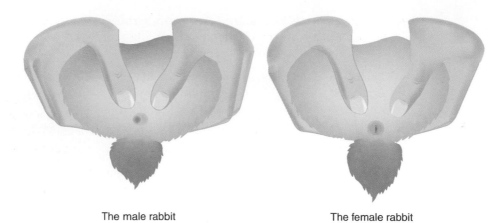

The male rabbit   The female rabbit

Fig. 17.5 Sexing rabbits. Source: Adapted from Ferris, M. (2003) Pet Store Management Course Manual. Reproduced with permission of The Pet Charity.

Sexing rabbits

Adult rabbits can be sexed quite easily but determination of sex in young rabbits can be difficult. Figure 17.5 shows the difference between the appearance of the genitals in a male and female rabbit.

Housing rabbits

There are many texts providing plans and layouts for both inside and outside housing. They also provide construction details for housing and runs and safe materials to use. It is important to ensure that any housing is of the right size for the eventual size of the adult rabbit and allow sufficient head clearance space for the rabbit to sit up on its hind legs. Rabbits and guinea pigs of similar size can be kept together, but this is a concept that is continually debated, and the animals must be monitored carefully to ensure that there is no bullying from either animal species (Fig. 17.6a). Figure 17.6b and c show enriched housing for individual species.

Rabbits do need regular exercise, ideally in an enclosed section of grass in the garden or a mobile run or in an assault course with wide plastic pipes in the hutch area. Logs (safe for rabbits) can be included in both run and hutch to add interest.

Housing for rabbits should:

- Protect from extremes of heat, cold and draughts. The preferred temperature is 12–20°C
- Be well constructed from good-quality materials. If materials have been treated, check that the chemicals used are non-toxic
- Be the correct size, with separate compartments for living and sleeping
- Protect from predators by being raised and fitted with a sturdy catch/lock system

- Contain materials for gnawing to reduce the teeth length. A supply of bark-covered logs from non-toxic trees (i.e. fruit trees) should be regularly changed
- Include an escape-proof portable outdoor 'summer' run for natural grazing and exercise
- Provide good ventilation
- Be easy to clean. Remove all soiled bedding on a daily basis and carry out a full clean on a weekly basis. Rabbits tend to use one spot in the hutch as a toilet and can be trained to use a cat litter tray. Ideal types of bedding include wood shavings to absorb urine and straw and hay for warmth. Disinfect at least monthly to remove the scale and odour from housing

(a)

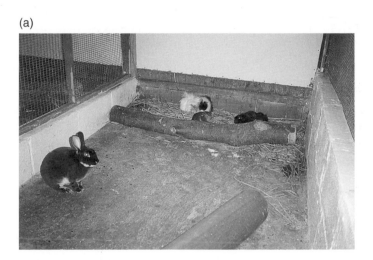

(b)

(c)

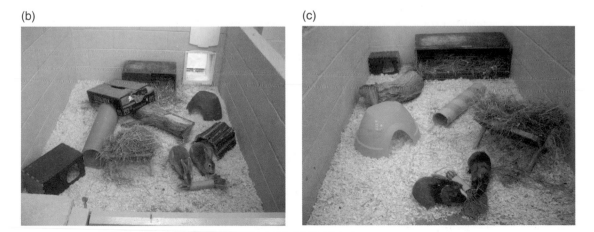

Fig. 17.6 (a) Example of group housing of rabbit and guinea pig. (b) Enriched rabbit-only housing. (c) Enriched guinea pig-only housing.

Feeding rabbits

Many rabbits are fed on commercially produced pelleted foods which may contain anti-coccidial agents which could be harmful to some species. Check the packaging if rabbits and guinea pigs feed together as these additives would be harmful to the guinea pig.

Rabbits are herbivores, so the main diet should consist of roughage: good-quality hay or grass, supplemented by herbs, leafy greens and vegetables. Select vegetables and greens carefully. Do not feed if any of the following are suspected or present:

- Greens are not freshly picked
- Mould is visible
- The feed is frozen or unwashed
- The feed has been sprayed with chemicals or weedkillers
- Plants that may be poisonous (see following text)

When selecting and feeding greens and vegetables, ensure that they are as fresh as possible and pesticide- and herbicide-free.

Muesli-type (cereal-based) foods were once popular as diets for rabbits, but it is now known that these should not be fed as they can cause dental and digestive problems in the rabbit as well as provide potential for selective feeding which can then lead to an unbalanced diet being eaten. Complete foods are similar to the rabbit mixes but with the addition of alfalfa to balance the cereals and provide the required dietary fibre content. These foods are useful for rabbits living in cities where there is no access to weeds, vegetation or hay.

Rabbit treats are manufactured commercially to exercise teeth; however, it is still important to provide natural sources, such as hay and twigs, to encourage gnawing to wear down the constantly growing teeth.

Some wild plants are poisonous to rabbits and should never be used for feed; these include:

- Any flowers or leaves from bulbs, i.e. tulip, bluebell or crocus
- Lily of the valley, laburnum or lupins
- Buttercups
- Deadly nightshade
- Scarlet pimpernel
- Bracken
- Hemlock (easily confused with hedge parsley)
- Foxglove
- Privet or yew
- Bindweed

Fresh water must be available at all times, from a water bottle and spout or a drinking bowl. If water bottles are used, the spout must be of a non-chewable material. Water bowls can be difficult to keep free of hay, food and droppings. Whichever method is used, a change of water must be made daily.

Guinea pigs

Guinea pigs (*Cavia porcellus*) are also known as 'cavies', and they belong to the order Rodentia, suborder Hystricomorpha, which also includes chinchillas, degus and porcupines to name a few other species. There are three main coat types of guinea pig, within which there are many colour and marking variations. These can be grouped as:

- Smooth or short hair (also referred to as self varieties), e.g. Self Golden or Dutch
- Containing whirls, ridges and rosettes, e.g. Abyssinian
- Long coated (up to 50 cm in length) with long, straight hairs, e.g. Peruvian, Texel and Sheltie. This type requires a lot of grooming and is mostly kept for showing, therefore not recommended for beginners

Guinea pigs can be nervous animals but are popular pets. They are generally docile, rarely bite, and are easy to handle and tame. They should not be kept on their own because they are very sociable animals. All-female or all-male groups can live together; however, the males must not be housed anywhere near the females as once they are sexually mature they will fight for dominance. Females and males can be neutered if non-breeding mixed groups are to be kept as pets.

Guinea pigs are not as agile as many of the other rodents, but they are able to run quite quickly, especially when startled, despite their short legs and stocky bodies. To communicate, guinea pigs are capable of making a range of noises, from squeaks and squeals to grunts. Guinea pigs are also known for their 'chattering'. Although guinea pigs do not dig, they are at home in dense undergrowth and enjoy making 'runs' through long grass. The main difference between the cavy and other rodents is the length of gestation and the resulting advanced stage of their young at birth.

Biological data: Guinea pigs

Male	Boar
Female	Sow
Offspring	Piglets
Adult weight	75–100 g
Maturity	Males: 8–10 weeks
	Females: 4–5 weeks
Gestation period	60–72 days
Litter size	2–6 (average size)
Weaning age	3–4 weeks
Body temperature	38–39°C
Life span	4–7 years

Anatomical facts: Guinea pigs

Teeth

- Dental formula: incisors 1/1, canines 0/0 (diastema), premolars 1/1 and molars 3/3.
- The teeth of a guinea pig are open rooted and chisel shaped, continuing to grow throughout its lifetime. Guinea pigs do not have the second small pair of incisors (peg teeth) found behind the main pair in rabbits; however, they do have a gap behind the incisors called the diastema. This allows the sides of the cheeks to be drawn in behind the incisors, enabling the animal to continue gnawing while regulating what it swallows.

Tail

- Born without a tail.

Scent glands

- Sebaceous glands are located on the rump and used to mark territory. In older animals, these glands can become blocked and infected, and this is something to watch out for.

Pelvis The pubic symphysis (floor of the pelvic joint) will separate under the influence of hormones during parturition, in order to allow the newborn passage through the birth canal. Newborn guinea pigs are referred to as *precocious*, meaning that within a few hours of birth, they are self-sufficient, eating and drinking from feeding dishes. They are born with a complete coat, with eyes and ears open and with a set of teeth in place.

Housing guinea pigs

Guinea pigs are sociable and can be housed as a colony. A single animal can be housed with another species such as a rabbit breed of similar size (see Fig. 17.6a) although there are different viewpoints in existence about this. Guinea pigs can be housed inside or outside providing it is a sheltered environment.

Housing should:

- Protect from extremes of temperature in summer and winter, similar to the rabbit
- Protect the animal from getting wet and exposure to draughts
- Be well constructed from good-quality materials which have not been treated with any toxic chemicals
- Be the correct size with separate compartments for eating and sleeping; rabbit housing can accommodate two to three guinea pigs

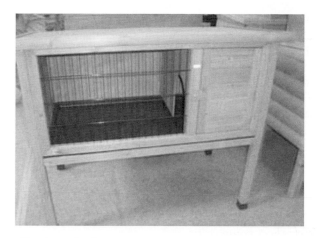

Fig. 17.7 Type of hutch used in housing.

- Provide good airflow and ventilation
- Protect from predators by being raised and fitted with a sturdy catch/lock system
- Contain materials for gnawing to reduce the teeth length. A supply of bark-covered logs from non-toxic trees (i.e. fruit trees) should be regularly changed
- Have a summer run for natural grazing or wire off a part of the garden to allow for space and freedom to exercise. Ideally, this run will be portable to allow movement onto different areas of grass. Be careful not to place the run in direct sunlight and provide a shaded area
- Be easy to clean. Use similar bedding as that used for rabbits, but it must be clean, dry and dust-free. Ideal types of bedding include wood shavings to absorb urine and straw and hay for warmth. Guinea pigs tend not to toilet in one area, so more frequent cleaning is required than for the rabbit. If feeding and water bowls are used, these need daily washing as they tend to be fouled
- Disinfect at least monthly to remove the scale and odour from housing.

An example of guinea pig housing is shown in Fig. 17.7.

Feeding guinea pigs

Guinea pigs are herbivores and spend most of their waking hours grazing if allowed. By nature, guinea pigs dislike any change to their routines, so watch for correct use of water feeders, if any changes have been made to the equipment. Guinea pigs often chew feed and water containers, and so choose metal or ceramic containers rather than plastic ones. A water bottle is better for providing water to a guinea pig than a bowl.

Commercially available pelleted guinea pig feed can be used. If any other prepared diet is used, then it is essential to supplement vitamin C, as ascorbic acid, in the diet, for skin and coat condition. *Guinea pigs are unable to manufacture vitamin C and must receive it in their diet.* Although some vitamin C can be obtained from natural grazing, they must have a daily supply of 10 mg/kg body weight. During pregnancy, the quantity of vitamin C can be increased by three times the normal daily amount to maintain a healthy animal.

Rabbit diets are generally not suitable for guinea pigs as they may contain levels of vitamin D that are too high for the guinea pig. Read the packaging and ask the supplier for advice. Supply good-quality roughage such as hay or cut grass. Supplement pelleted food with fresh vegetables (swedes and carrots) and fruits. Useful green foods include broccoli, dandelion and groundsel. Always provide fresh drinking water daily, using similar drinking bottles and spouts to those found in rabbit housing.

Handling guinea pigs

Handling of guinea pigs should be carried out quietly and confidently to avoid unnecessary struggling which could result in injury to the guinea pig or to the handler. Talk quietly to the guinea pig in a reassuring voice to minimize any distress. As long as guinea pigs feel secure throughout the whole handling process, there should be no problems.

When lifting a guinea pig, it is important to be gentle:

- Place one hand over the guinea pig's shoulders and back, and using the other hand to support the back end of the guinea pig, lift the guinea pig up.
- Once lifted, a guinea pig should be turned towards you so that it feels secure with its feet on your chest.
- Alternatively, a guinea pig can be cradled along the arm.
- A guinea pig will struggle if it does not feel secure, and this can cause injury to both the handler and the guinea pig.

Sexing guinea pigs

Once the technique is learnt, it is very easy to distinguish between the males and the females. The guinea pig should be lying supported on its back with its back legs facing away from you. Place gentle pressure on the lower abdomen in the genital area. In a male animal, the penis will be displayed. In females, a 'Y' shape tends to be observed (Fig. 17.8). Once guinea pigs have been sexed, they should be kept in separate groups if breeding is not required.

Mice

Mice kept as pets are known as fancy mice and are derived from the wild house mouse. Mice belong to the order Rodentia, suborder Myomorpha – *Mus musculus*.

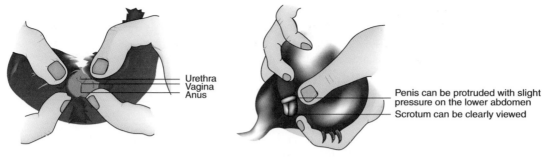

Female-seen as a "Y" shape

Urethra
Vagina
Anus

Penis can be protruded with slight
pressure on the lower abdomen
Scrotum can be clearly viewed

Male-penis can be protruded with pressure

Fig. 17.8 Sexing guinea pigs. Source: Adapted from Ferris, M. (2003) Pet Store Management Course Manual. Reproduced with permission of The Pet Charity.

They are initially categorised according to their coat type (varieties), and then, they are grouped into sections within each variety according to their colour and body markings. Varieties include long hairs, Rex and Satins.

Mice are very social animals and must live either as a breeding pair or in a grouping of two or more females, but male mice will fight if kept together. Mice have a very high reproductive rate, and so a pair should only be kept together if you can guarantee homes for the offspring. Mice are very agile and quick to move. They can make good pets and are lively, friendly, intelligent and inquisitive animals. Mice are fairly easy to tame and rarely bite unless threatened. Aggression is signalled by drumming the tail on the ground and stamping the hind legs. They are efficient climbers, clinging to surfaces and clothing of handlers, making handling easy. Mice do tend to be more active at night, communicating with each other by body language and voice, squeaking (high-frequency, high-pitch sounds) when frightened. Odour can be a problem, particularly with male animals, and so it is important to clean them out at least once a week.

Biological data: Mice

Male	Buck
Female	Doe
Offspring	Kittens/pups
Adult weight	20–40 g
Maturity	3–4 weeks
Gestation period	19–21 days
Litter size	5–11 (average size)
Weaning age	18 days
Body temperature	37.5°C
Life span	1–2.5 years

Anatomical facts

Teeth

- Dental formula: incisors 1/1, canines 0/0, premolars 0/0 and molars 3/3.
- A mouse's teeth are open rooted and continue to grow (incisor teeth only). The lower jaw is also adapted in movement to allow gnawing or chewing.

Eyes

- Vision is not good, but because of the eye position (on the side of the head), the field of vision compensates. As a result, mice navigate their environment through smell and touch. Mice see better at night than in the day.

Feet

- Using scent glands on the soles of their feet, they can mark territory and food location.

Housing mice

The best accommodation for mice is a glass tank of at least 1200 cm² area and approximately 60 cm deep with a close fitting wire mesh lid to prevent condensation from building up. Mice enjoy climbing and so need relatively tall cages. Alternatively, mice can be kept in wire cages as they will enjoy climbing on the bars around the cage but ensure the bars are narrow so that the mice cannot escape through them. Plastic cages are easy to clean but are chewable.

It is important that any housing for mice is environmentally enriched with tubes, ropes, exercise wheels and compartments. Plenty of enrichment will enable the mouse to exercise and keep busy to maintain health and fitness (Fig. 17.9).

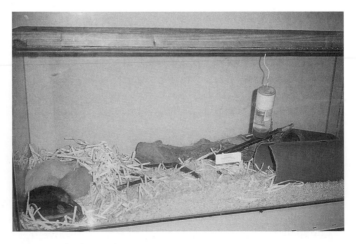

Fig. 17.9 Housing with plenty of compartments.

Housing for mice should:

- Be escape proof, using commercial metal, glass or plastic cages or tanks
- Be kept indoors, with an activity area and nest box containing a variety of bedding materials (shredded paper, hay or straw)
- Have no direct sunlight or draughts, thus avoiding extremes of temperature. Mice are best kept at 15–27°C/59–81°F. If the temperature rises above 30°C, then the mice can suffer from heat stroke
- Be dry and easy to clean
- Be cleaned at least once a week, preferably twice a week to reduce odour and accumulation of urine and faeces
- Contain plenty of enrichment
- Contain materials for gnawing to promote good tooth condition. Gnaw blocks may be bought from pet shops, or natural non-toxic branches such as apple twigs may be used instead

Feeding mice

- Mice are omnivores.
- Diets in pellet form are available which are balanced in the nutrition required by the mouse. Mice require some animal-based protein in their diet, which the commercial foods will provide. They benefit from other additions to the diet, such as small quantities of dog biscuit, wholemeal bread, pieces of fruit (apples, grapes and strawberries) and vegetables (especially green vegetables) in small amounts, several times a week. If peanuts and sunflower seeds are given, monitor their intake as they can be fattening for the mouse due to their high lipid content. Too much fruit will result in diarrhoea.
- A mouse will eat approximately 3–6 g of food/day. Mice will store their food and so it is necessary to check for uneaten food that may go mouldy. Remove any uneaten food materials each morning.
- Food bowls may be provided and should be made of metal or ceramic so that the mice do not chew them. Alternatively, it is better to scatter feed for enrichment purposes.
- Water must be provided at all times, via a water bottle and sipper tube. Ensure the bottle is suspended above the level of the substrate or the dispensing spout will become blocked. Fresh water should be provided on a daily basis.

Handling mice

Scoop the mouse up in cupped hands or lift by the **base** of the tail and place onto outstretched palm for stability and security. For an individual mouse that is difficult to catch, aim to coax it into a small pot to remove from the tank before trying to pick it up.

To restrain the mouse, place the forefinger and thumb of one hand on either side of the mouse's head to keep the head still and cup the body of the mouse in the hand.

Sexing mice

An adult male mouse will be easy to sex due to the obvious visual presence of testicles. However, the most reliable method to use is to examine the distance between the anus and the urethral opening. In a male, there is a longer distance between the two. Younger mice are more difficult to sex, but females are likely to have more obvious nipple presence.

Rats

Rats kept as pets are also known as fancy rats. Belonging to the order Rodentia and sub-order Myomorpha, the fancy rat species is from the wild brown rat, *Rattus norvegicus*. They are categorized first according to their coat type (varieties, e.g. hooded or selfs) and then grouped into sections by colour and body markings. Varieties available include albinos, hooded, Rex and Siamese.

Rats are very social animals and will happily live together although they can be kept on their own if they have plenty of human attention. Rats can be housed as breeding pairs or groups of the same sex although adult males may fight after puberty. Rats are highly intelligent and so require plenty of enrichment. They can be trained to respond to their name and learn a variety of tricks. Unlike other rodents, they need at least an hour a day of play time outside their cage or housing. A single rat would require more.

Rats can make good pets for older children. They are good climbers and very inquisitive. They make little noise, but odour can be a problem, particularly if groups of males are kept together, and so they must be cleaned out once a week as a minimum.

Biological data: Rats

Male	Buck
Female	Doe
Offspring	Pups
Adult weight	400–800 g
Maturity	6 weeks onwards
Gestation period	20–22 days
Litter size	6–12 (average size)
Weaning age	21 days
Body temperature	38°C
Life span	3 years

Anatomical facts: Rats

Teeth

- Dental formula: incisors 1/1, canines 0/0, premolars 0/0 and molars 3/3.
- Rats have open-rooted incisor teeth which continue to grow throughout their life.

Long bones

- Ossify in the second year of life. This means that under 1 year of age, their bones are quite soft.

Digestive tract

- Rats have a divided stomach, large caecum and no gall bladder.

Housing rats

The best accommodation for rats is a chinchilla or chipmunk cage that allows for plenty of exercise. Rats enjoy climbing and so need relatively tall cages. Rats will live in small groups or alone, but do need plenty of space for activity, toys and environmental enrichment. They can become attached to their owners, are quick to learn and are easy to train. Rats will burrow given the opportunity and can be nocturnal.

Housing should:

- Provide enough space for a nest box and activity areas
- Be inside but not in direct sunlight or draughts. Rats are best kept at 15–27°C/59–81°F. If the temperature rises too high, then the rats can suffer from heat stroke
- Rats should be provided with toys, as they like to spend a lot of time investigating equipment and exploring their enclosure. Toilet rolls and large plastic pipes make good toys for rats as well as wooden toys, knotted ropes, ladders, etc. Non-toxic branches are excellent for allowing the rats to climb in their cage. The environment should be interesting, with different levels (Figs. 17.10 and 17.11)
- Be easy to clean and be cleaned two to three times per week to reduce odour, urine and faeces. Use a dust-free, absorbent litter in the cage, with shredded paper for bedding in the nest area
- Have a solid floor to avoid injury to the rat's feet
- Be gnaw proof and made of materials not treated with toxic chemicals
- It is vital that substances for gnawing are provided for the rat in order to keep their teeth in good condition. Gnaw blocks may be bought from pet shops, or natural non-toxic branches such as apple twigs may be used instead

Feeding rats

- Rats are omnivores.
- Diets can be bought in pellet form and these contain a balanced diet for the rat. The protein content of the food should be between 25% and 40%. The rat diet can be

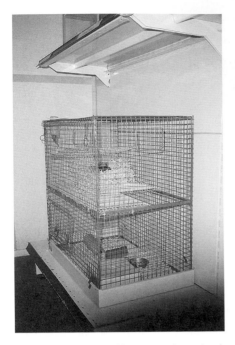

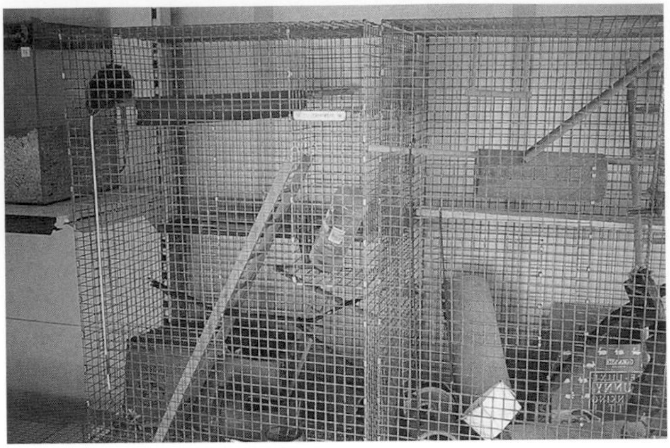

Fig. 17.11 Close-up view of a two-level house.

Fig. 17.10 Type of housing with two levels for a rat.

added to in the form of lean meat scraps from the table or dog food, wholegrain cereals, fruits and some vegetables. If sunflower seeds or peanuts are given, then the amount should be monitored as they are fattening due to their high lipid content and so should not be given in excess.

- Rats do not eat strange or new foods readily.
- Provide fresh water daily, using a bottle and sipper tube to prevent contamination. Ensure it is suspended above the level of the substrate or the dispensing spout will become blocked.
- Rats will eat approximately 25 g of food/day.
- Food bowls may be provided and should be made of metal or ceramic so that the rats do not chew them. Alternatively, it is better to scatter feed to enrich their environment.

Handling rats

Rats can be lifted up across their shoulders or they can be scooped up, or when young, they can be lifted by the **base** of the tail and placed onto outstretched palm for stability.

To restrain the rat, place the forefinger and thumb of one hand on either side of the rat's head to keep the head still and support the body of the rat in the other hand unless it is small enough to cup in the same hand that is holding the head still.

Sexing rats

An adult male rat will be easy to sex due to the obvious visual presence of testicles. However, the most reliable method to use is to examine the distance between the anus and the urethral opening. In a male, there is a longer distance between the two. Younger rats are more difficult to sex, but females are likely to have more obvious nipple presence as in mice.

Hamsters

Hamsters are one of the most popular small pets. Belonging to the order Rodentia, sub-order Myomorpha, there are over 20 species of hamster. However, those most commonly kept as pets are:

- *Syrian (golden) hamster – (Mesocricetus auratus)* – must be kept singly as adults. They are aggressive to other hamsters, both male and female, once they reach puberty. They are known to hibernate if their environmental temperature falls below 5°C. There is a wide range of colours of Syrian hamster available, and they are referred to as individual breeds, e.g. black-eyed cream, Swedish Black and Cinnamon. Coat types also contribute to different hamster breeds, e.g. Satins and long hairs
- *Russian hamsters – (Phodopus sungorus)* – the most sociable of all the hamsters. In the wild, they live in family groups rather than alone. They should preferably be kept in pairs or as small groups, and if not handled regularly, they can become aggressive. They have a similar shape to the Syrian hamster but are much smaller. Colours include cinnamon, grey, sapphire and spotted and winter white
- *Chinese hamsters – (Cricetulus griseus)* – less sociable than the Russian hamster but can be kept in pairs or small groups if introduced to each other when young. They are slightly smaller in size than the Russian hamster but have a longer body with a small visible tail
- *Roborovski hamsters – (Phodopus roborovskii)* – are the smallest of all the hamsters. They resemble a Russian hamster in appearance with a white moustache. The Roborovski is not recommended as a pet for children because it is so small and active and therefore hard to handle

Hamsters are active at dawn and dusk (referred to as *crepuscular* animals) but sleep most of the day. Dwarf hamsters tend to show more activity during the day. Hamsters are escapologists and any cage needs to be secure. During their travels, they can cover up to 11 km. Dwarf hamsters, such as the very small Roborovski hamster, are best kept in tanks or cages sold as mouse housing. Hamsters can bite if disturbed from sleep, and when feeling threatened or aggressive, they sometimes squeal, screech or hiss. They live according to smell, becoming accustomed to the scent of the group if not living singly. If one animal has been handled extensively or placed in the company of another, the group may attack it.

Biological data: Hamsters

	Syrian (golden)	**Chinese**	**Russian**
Male	Sire	Sire	Sire
Female	Dam	Dam	Dam
Offspring	Pups	Pups	Pups
Adult weight	85–150 g	27–35 g	27–35 g
Maturity	6–10 weeks	14 weeks	14 weeks
Gestation period	15–18 days	20–22 days	19–20 days
Litter size	3–7	3–7	3–7
Weaning age	21–28 days	20–22 days	20–22 days
Body temperature	37–38°C	37–38°C	37–38°C
Life span	1.5–2 years	1.5–2 years	1.5–2 years

Anatomical facts: Hamsters

Teeth

- Incisors are open rooted and continually grow. They must be regularly checked to ensure they are not overgrown.
- Dental formula: incisors 1/1, canines 0/0, premolars 0/0 and molars 3/3.

Mouth

- Hamsters have large cheek pouches, reaching almost to the scapula area of the shoulder, used to transport food or store it temporarily.

Eyes

- Hamsters are short sighted and rely on scent within their enclosure.

Scent glands

- Situated in the flank region and used to mark territory, these are seen as darker patches of skin and are also known as *flank glands*. They can be obvious in older animals leading owners to think there is skin problem.

Housing hamsters

Syrian hamsters are naturally solitary animals, tending to fight in group situations. Dwarf hamsters will happily live in pairs or small groups if raised together from a young age. When awake, hamsters have a lot of energy. Hamsters in the wild will dig tunnels close to the surface.

There is a wide variety of accommodation available for hamsters. Hamster housing should be as big as possible so that the hamster can gain adequate exercise. Hamsters need plenty of living space and a smaller area for sleeping. A rough size guide is 2400 cm^2 × 30 cm high.

To prevent boredom, housing should include playthings such as cardboard tubes, empty jam jars and exercise wheels of a solid construction. If the temperature of their environment drops below 5°C, hibernation for survival may occur, particularly with the Syrian hamster.

Hamsters will chew soft metals, plastic and wood, and so it is best to avoid these materials in the housing if possible.

Hamster housing should:

- Be constructed from materials that are nonabsorbent, easy to clean and relatively non-chewable
- Have side access to the cage so that the hamster doesn't think that the owner/carer is a predator and so attack them
- Have only safe bedding materials, such as peat or wood shavings as a base, covered with untreated paper or cardboard for shredding and nesting
- Be kept inside
- Not be in direct sunlight. The temperature should be approximately 22°C. Remember, hamsters may try to hibernate if the temperature drops too low
- Be well ventilated but not draughty
- Include a sleeping house
- Be cleaned at least two to three times a week
- Provide exercise equipment, such as a wheel, tunnels, ladders and plenty of safe materials for shredding
- Bedding – wood shavings can be used in the bottom of the cage and shredded paper for the resting area. Hay should not be used as it can damage the hamster's pouches. Nylon bed material should not be used as it can get twisted around the hamster's legs and also get stuck in their pouches, and this can cause them to become infected

Feeding hamsters

- Hamsters are relatively easy animals to feed although a lot of hamsters are overweight due to a lack of exercise and being given too much food.
- The hamster is an omnivore and can be fed a commercially produced 'hamster mix' food, which contains maize, corn, alfalfa, dried peas, sunflower seeds and peanuts. The diet should contain some animal protein, such as small quantities of cat and dog food or raw meat (not pork). Vegetables and fruits (e.g. carrot, apple) will help to improve health status, with small quantities given daily. Hamsters need a supply of food to gnaw in order to prevent incisor overgrowth. As well as the nuts in the diet, dog biscuits and wholemeal macaroni can be provided.
- Hamsters will attempt to eat and hoard anything; therefore, they must not be given cake or sweets. The adult hamster will eat its own droppings, particularly for vitamins B and K formed in the gut by bacteria.

- Food can be provided on an *ad-lib* basis for hamsters, but the bowl should not be filled up until the bowl is empty so that the hamster does not become fussy. Check for areas of stored food in the housing and clean them up before re-filling the bowl.
- Provide fresh drinking water daily using a water bottle and sipper tube. Ensure the bottle is suspended where the hamster can reach it and out of the way of the substrate so the dispensing tube does not become blocked.

Handling hamsters

Once a hamster is awake, let it explore its surroundings and come to you. Stroke a hamster first so it gets used to your smell. Do not rush a hamster or it may bite. Either let the hamster climb into the handler's hand, scoop it up in cupped hands or in an object of some description or place one hand firmly over its shoulders and back and lift into the other hand (Fig. 17.12). Once picked up, let the hamster wander between the handler's hands. In order to restrain a hamster, place the thumb and forefinger to either side of the head and hold still or scruff gently at the back of the neck. Never handle a hamster or scruff a hamster that has full cheek pouches – allow them to empty them first.

It is important to be confident when handling hamsters as they are able to sense nervousness and will bite. Regular handling is good for hamsters as it gets them used to humans.

Sexing hamsters

- Male and female hamsters are sexually mature at an early age and so should be separated from 6 weeks of age.
- Adult hamsters are relatively easy to sex as when viewed from the above; the male has a more pointed look to the back end of his body due to the presence of testicles. In females, the end of their body is more rounded although the tail can look more prominent.
- Young hamsters are not so easy to sex, but it can be done by observing the distance between the anus and the genital areas – in males, the distance is greater than in females (Fig. 17.13).

Gerbils

The species most commonly kept as a pet is the Mongolian gerbil – *Meriones unguiculatus*. Gerbils belong to the order Rodentia, suborder Myomorpha, and there are about 80 species of gerbil in the wild. The gerbil is adapted to living in desert and semi-desert areas (Mongolia and northeastern China).

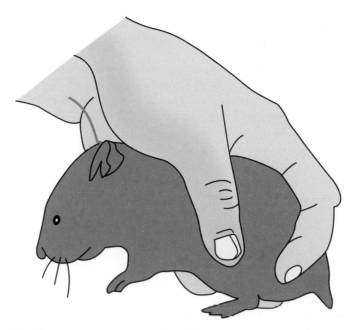

Fig. 17.12 Handling a hamster. Source: Adapted from Ferris, M. (2003) Pet Store Management Course Manual. Reproduced with permission of The Pet Charity.

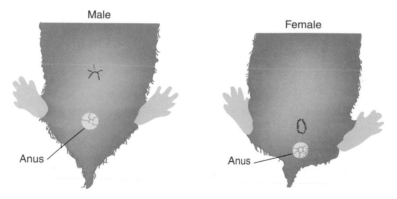

Fig. 17.13 Sexing hamsters. Source: Adapted from Ferris, M. (2003) Pet Store Management Course Manual. Reproduced with permission of The Pet Charity.

As a result of their wild habitat, gerbils can conserve liquid, producing very concentrated urine and dry faeces, which are odour-free. Gerbils are camouflaged in the wild due to their beige coat colour and reflect heat from their pale underneath to keep cool.

Gerbils are active both day and night (referred to as *diurnal*). In body proportions, the gerbil closely resembles the kangaroo, jumping rather than running when attacked. In the wild, gerbils can leap several feet in any direction, especially if startled, which, as a pet, can make them hard to handle although with sufficient handling, they become friendly.

Gerbils are lively, intelligent and inquisitive animals. They sit up on their hind legs to watch for predators and communicate danger through thumping their hind legs or indicate their dominance. They spend a large part of their day burrowing, shredding bedding, tunnelling and exploring. They love to burrow and so need a soft, deep substrate to build tunnels and create nests.

Gerbils are very social animals and are best kept together in groups, with same-sex litter mates or in breeding pairs. Gerbils will mate for life and should be introduced around 10 weeks of age. Adult gerbils will fight to the death so try not to introduce adults to a stable family group.

Biological data

Male	Sire
Female	Dam
Offspring	Cubs
Adult weight	75–130 kg (depending on breed)
Maturity	10–12 weeks
Gestation period	24–28 days
Litter size	3–6 (average size)
Weaning age	21–28 days
Body temperature	38°C
Life span	2–5 years (average)

Anatomical facts: Gerbils

Teeth

- Incisors are open rooted and continue to grow through the gerbil's life. Check regularly.
- Dental formula: incisors 1/1, canines 0/0, premolars 0/0 and molars 3/3.

Scent glands

- Gerbils have scent glands on their abdomen, which are used for identification of members of the same family and marking of territory.

Adrenal glands

- Hormones from these endocrine glands assist the gerbil's ability to conserve water in adverse conditions.

Hind legs

- Longer than front legs; therefore, they can jump to escape from predators.

Tail

- Used for balance and turning.
- Gerbils have a dark tip on the end of their tail which acts as a decoy for predators. The tail can be shed if the gerbil is in danger or if it is grasped away from its base, but it does not re-grow.

Eyes

- Gerbils have relatively large eyes and very good vision.

Hearing

- Gerbils have an acute sense of hearing due to an enlarged middle ear in order to hear birds flying above and avoid being eaten.

Housing gerbils

Gerbils are social animals and will live in groups but can be aggressive to any newcomer. As pets, they are easy to handle, clean and friendly.

Gerbils are adapted to live in extremes of temperature, from 43°C to below freezing. The gerbil is a burrowing animal, creating elaborate tunnel systems and entrances. They do this to find a constant temperature within the ground. The burrowing material, peat, hay or wood shavings, needs to be dampened slightly to allow tunnels to be constructed that keep their shape. Sand must not be used on its own as a substrate as it may cause eye problems or respiratory problems. Shredded paper or hay can be provided so that the gerbil can build a nest/bed area.

The ideal housing is a glass tank of at least 90 cm in length, approximately 30 cm deep, with a close fitting mesh lid. Allow enough room between the lid and the tunnel material for above-ground or surface activity and prevent condensation.

Gerbil housing should:

- Be escape proof
- Contain only non-toxic materials, as gerbils will gnaw anything in their environment
- Be in a warm environment; 18–29°C is ideal. Gerbils are best kept at 15–20°C/ 59–68°F. Gerbils do not hibernate
- Be washed, disinfected and rinsed every 2 months
- It is vital that substances for gnawing are provided for the gerbil in order to keep their teeth in good condition. Gnaw blocks may be bought from pet shops, or alternatively, natural non-toxic branches such as apple twigs may be used instead. Putting branches in the cage also allows the gerbil to get exercise by climbing, but ensure that they are not too near to the roof or they may escape
- Have good light levels in the daytime to encourage activity

- Gerbils may occasionally be provided with a dust bath filled with chinchilla sand, as they like to take a 'bath' to help keep their coats in good condition
- Gerbils produce only a few drops of urine and faecal pellets are dry and odourless, so bedding only needs to be changed about every 2–4 weeks, unless it is particularly dirty

Feeding gerbils

The gerbil is an omnivore, but its diet includes grain (such as wheat, maize, oats, barley), seeds (such as millet, sunflower) and greens (such as lettuce, dandelion, groundsel, chickweed). Sunflower seeds should be restricted as these are too rich in fat and calcium, which can lead to dietary imbalance and ill health. An animal protein source may be included in a commercial gerbil food, or table scraps or boiled egg can be added to the diet. The protein content of the food should be approximately 20%. Also, supplement the diet with fresh fruits and vegetables, such as apple, banana and carrot, but be careful not to overfeed or this can cause diarrhoea.

A gerbil will eat approximately 1 tablespoonful of food/day. The gerbil will hoard food in a larger area of its housing. Always remove the uneaten food to prevent it becoming stale. It is better to scatter feed the food as an enrichment, but if bowls are provided, then they should be metal or ceramic so that gerbils cannot chew them.

Water must be supplied in bottles with dispensing spouts. The bottles can be attached to the side of the tank or the lid, but ensure it is suspended above the level of the substrate or the dispensing spout will become blocked. The water should be supplied fresh daily.

Handling gerbils

To handle a gerbil, it is better to scoop it up in cupped hands or an appropriate container. Do not attempt to lift a gerbil by the tail as it may be shed which will cause pain to the gerbil.

Birds

Birds are kept either as pets, for breeding or for exhibition. They can be housed singly in cages of suitable size or in groups in large outdoor aviaries. There are many different species of bird (class: Aves), which are assigned to 27 orders.

The orders most commonly seen are:

- Anseriformes – ducks, geese and swans
- Falconiformes – diurnal hawks and falcons
- Galliformes – domestic fowl and pheasants
- Passeriformes – finches and canaries (passerines) (Fig. 17.14)

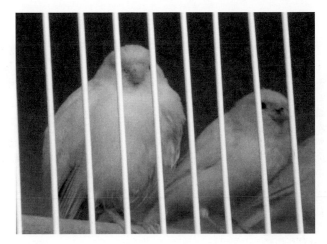

Fig. 17.14 Canaries.

- Psittaciformes – parrots and budgerigars (psittacines)
- Strigiformes – owls
- Columbiformes – pigeons and doves

Most pet cage birds come from one of two main orders:

- Passerines – perching birds (e.g. canary, finch)
- Psittacines – climbing birds (e.g. budgerigar)

The two main features of anatomy which distinguish these two groups are:

- beak conformation – passerines peck at seeds, whereas psittacines open fruit and nuts
- foot conformation – passerines have three outer toes facing forwards and one inner toe facing backwards (Fig. 17.15), whereas psittacines have two middle toes facing forwards and two outer toes facing backwards (Fig. 17.16)

Other anatomical facts

- *Skeleton* – bones are thin, some containing air sacs (linked to the respiratory system) making up a lightweight structure for flight.
- *Digestive tract* – food is stored in the crop; the gizzard then grinds the food to pass to the intestines. The opening cloaca is a common end to the outside for the digestive, urinary and reproductive tracts.
- *Respiratory system* – birds have no diaphragm; the lungs are set out in pairs through the thorax and abdomen area (Fig. 17.17). The bird's respiratory system is complex for improved flow of air to the tissues.

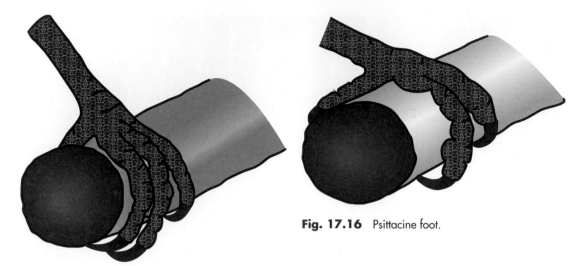

Fig. 17.16 Psittacine foot.

Fig. 17.15 Passerine foot.

For many pet owners, their choice is the budgerigar. Belonging to the parakeet family of birds, budgerigars have a chattering call and can be taught words and simple tunes. They are easy to keep, both in housing and feeding needs. If budgerigars are let out of their housing into a room, they will normally return to the accommodation quite readily. Some birds are valued for their song, such as the canary (particularly the male bird). Canaries belong to the finch family of birds, which are quick moving, hard to catch and usually kept in an aviary-type housing and as a group.

If pet birds do share the house uncaged, it is important to remember that birds like to explore and should not be left unattended. Precautions to take before letting the bird out of its cage include:

- Close all windows and doors
- Do not allow flight or access to the kitchen area, because of hot surfaces and fumes fatal to a bird
- Check that electrical cables are not exposed and that electrical fans are switched off
- Remove houseplants that are toxic to birds, such as cacti
- Remove other pets, such as dogs or cats

Housing for pet birds must be easily cleaned, both daily to remove droppings and, more thoroughly, monthly. Birds are kept as pets for many reasons, one of which is to display their beauty, achieved by keeping them in:

- Cages (Fig. 17.18)
- Aviaries

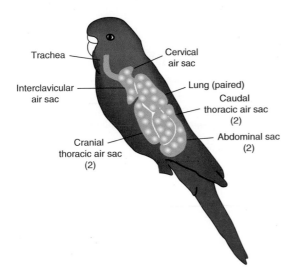

Fig. 17.17 Avian respiratory system.

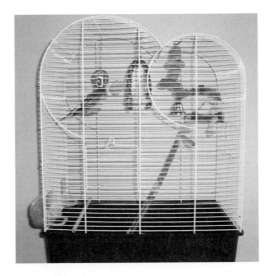

Fig. 17.18 Budgerigar cage type in common use.

Cage system

There are many types of cage available, with a variety of costs, size and design. However, many are unsuitable for the many varied species kept as pets. A cage should be as large as possible, especially if the bird is going to be confined for much of the day in it.

A bird cage must:

- Be large enough to allow the bird to stretch its wings up and out without touching the sides of the cage
- Not cause the bird to fly in an artificial way, i.e. circular cages
- Be strong and well constructed with no sharp edges (especially around the cage base)
- Have safe cage fittings, i.e. materials that cannot be chewed used for food containers
- Have good door fastenings so that the bird(s) can't get out and nothing else can get in
- Be easy to keep clean
- Have meshwork or bars on one side to give a feeling of security to the bird
- Be placed well above the ground level, i.e. at eye height
- Provide environmental enrichment (toys/activities)
- Have a variety of perches (not covered with sand paper as these can damage the feet)
- Be sited away from draughts, direct sunlight and any harmful fumes (cooking fumes, i.e. over-heated oil, cigarette smoke and room sprays)
- Be cleaned daily (removal of unwanted fresh foods, seeds and droppings)

Aviary system

There are many advantages to pet birds when housed in a larger space such as an aviary. Flight becomes possible, providing a more natural environment, complete with plants and secluded areas. There are disadvantages as well. Aviaries are more difficult to clean as it is more time consuming to remove dropped foods, but this must be done to reduce the risk of disease being introduced to the pet birds by wild birds, mice and rats that are attracted by the uneaten foodstuff. The most obvious concern for birds housed outside is their exposure to cold and hot weather conditions.

An aviary must:

- Be well designed, with a safety door, as large as possible in size and high enough for good flight but be easy to clean
- Be made of materials that will cause no harm (to include gauge of the netting and wood types used)
- Have a floor/base that is easy to clean, i.e. concrete
- Have perches of different diameters and heights
- Have shallow baths or a misting system for bathing
- Be covered in part (or one entire side) to avoid wind and rain
- Have an inside shelter of boxes to encourage roosting at night
- Be secure to avoid bird escapes and entry by other species
- Ideally have a double door entry system
- Ensure a 12 hour period of daylight, using lighting systems in the winter, to encourage food intake in the correct amounts
- Never have food containers placed under perches; preferably, they should be off the floor

Budgerigars

The budgerigar (*Melopsittacus undulatus*) is available in a wide range of colours, but in the wild, it is green. It originates from Australia, where its natural habitat is semi-arid (hot) grassland with trees, near water holes. All budgies originated from the light-green variety found in the wild. Other colours started to appear late in the nineteenth century as birds showed an increase in popularity. Varieties include the Lutino, Grey Winged Sky Blue, Crested Opaline Cobalt, Grey, Recessive Pied Violet and Spangle Light Green.

Budgerigars are the most practical of the cage birds. They are lively, colourful, quite hardy and diurnal and can be brought up to mimic human speech. Although they need daily attention, they are reasonably cheap to house and feed.

Biological data

Male	Cock
Female	Hen
Offspring	Chick

Adult weight	30–35 g
Sexing	A male bird has blue cere
	A female has brown cere
Maturity	5 months onwards
Clutch	3–6 white eggs
Incubation time	18 days to hatch (up to 3 weeks)
Fledgling	Further 35 days
Body temperature	40–42°C
Life span	6–8 years

Anatomical facts

Beak

- This is a hinge joint between the skull and upper beak. With no teeth, this allows increased movements suitable for slicing through nut shells, with the help of a flexible tongue to obtain food (Fig. 17.19).

Feeding budgerigars

- Budgies are hard-billed birds and so eat seeds.
- Seed mixes containing various types of millet and linseed, fruit and occasional insects can be fed. It may be necessary to give or provide an iodine supplement if one is not already included in the seed mix given.
- Fresh fruits, vegetables and green foods (dandelion, chickweed, groundsel and lettuce) add interest and nutrients to the diet.
- Vitamin D must be supplemented if there is no access to sunlight.
- The seed and fruit should be given in bowls but do not place bowls directly under perches in order to prevent contamination with bird droppings.
- A supply of calcium as cuttlefish should be held in the cage clips for the bird to attack.
- Fresh water should be readily available from drinkers.
- Grit mixture (oyster shell and particles of stone/rock) should be available to aid digestion.

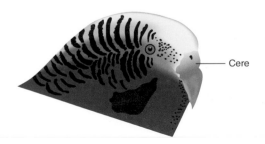

Cere

Fig. 17.19 Budgerigar beak.

- When feeding, blow husks off the top of the bowl to see how much feed is left.
- Food bowls should be metal or plastic not ceramic, as they get broken easily. Water containers should be cleaned thoroughly to prevent algal growth.

Handling budgerigars

Ensure all doors and windows are shut before attempting to catch the budgie. The method of catching will vary according to whether the bird is housed in an indoor cage or an outdoor aviary. A bird net may be needed in the latter case.

Once the bird has been caught, place one hand over the bird's back and use the thumb and forefinger on the same hand to restrain the head. Hold the bird firmly but gently to prevent struggling. If the bird is held too tightly, then it can suffocate.

It is important to keep the head still to prevent injury to the handler. A budgie can give a very hard bite – remember that the beak is designed to eat seeds!

Sexing budgerigars

Determining the sex of the bird is relatively easy in adult birds. Males have a blue cere and females have a brown/pink cere. Young birds have brown ceres. Alternatively, DNA sexing can occur.

Canaries

Canaries are found in a wide range of colours and markings but in the wild are in greenish-yellow colour only. The canary (*Serinus canaria*) is part of the finch family of birds and belongs to the order Passeriformes (passerines).

Canaries originate from the Canary Islands and parts of Europe. The natural habitat for the canary is scrubland, fields and pastures, and it is diurnal. Passerines are perching birds, best kept in aviary flocks because it is rare that they are tame enough to handle.

Biological data

Male	Cock
Female	Hen
Offspring	Chick
Adult weight	20 g
Sexing	When mature, both sexes look alike. The male bird song is the best. To be sure of obtaining a male, birds are usually bought several months after fledging, by which time the cock birds will be distinguished by their song
Clutch	3–6 eggs are laid every other day
Incubation time	14 days
Fledgling	Further 14 days
Body temperature	40–42°C
Life span	6–9 years

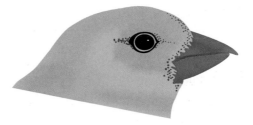

Fig. 17.20   Canary beak.

Anatomical fact

Beak

- This is short and conical in shape and used to crack seeds when feeding (Fig. 17.20).

Feeding canaries

- Canaries are hard-billed seed eaters. Their food contains both cereals and oil seeds such as canary seed, millet, rape seed and hemp. It is important to remove the husks from the feed container every day to enable feeding. Appropriately sized grit (soluble and insoluble) must be available in order to grind the seeds in the gizzard.
- Commercial complete diets are available, but some fresh green foods (lettuce, dandelion, chickweed and alfalfa), fruits and vegetables should also be offered.
- Remove any uneaten fresh foods or soaked seeds daily. Soaking enables germination of seeds, which improves the nutritional value, but it is important that these are well drained and removed after a few hours if not eaten to avoid fungal growth which could be harmful. Tonic foods, which include a greater range of seed types and are for occasional use, are also available commercially.
- Ensure a fresh supply of water, changed daily in the housing (cage or aviary), and thorough cleaning of the water containers to prevent growth of algae.

Fish

Fish make excellent pets, and in terms of numbers, they are the most commonly kept pet. Fish are attractive, colourful and interesting to study or just watch. Fish do not demand much time (depending on the complexity of the tank or the species kept) and do not make any noise. Feeding costs are relatively low and equipment can be reasonably simple or as elaborate and expensive as you wish to make it.

Types of fish commonly kept as pets fall into four main groups:

- Coldwater (10–26°C)
- Tropical freshwater (21–29°C)

- Tropical marine (21–29°C)
- Coldwater marine (10–26°C)

Of the three groups, coldwater and tropical freshwater fish are normally kept by pet owners and hobbyists. Tropical and coldwater marine fish are complex to keep, and a good understanding of their requirements is essential.

Marine fish live in sea water, and they are hypotonic (i.e. less salty than the sea water that is their environment); this causes water to be drawn out of these fish by osmosis (see Chapter 2). To counteract this dehydration, they must continuously take in water by drinking. The fish will die rapidly if the water they drink is not:

- Filtered of excretions (containing ammonia and nitrite)
- The same salt concentration and pH of sea water all the time

Anatomical data

External anatomical features

Fins (Fig. 17.21) give stability in the water, control the direction of movement and can be divided into:

- Single – tend to be dorsal (top fin for balance), adipose (in some fish only), caudal (tail fin for propelling forward) and anal (for balance)
- Paired – pectoral and ventral (pelvic fins) both used for steering
- Fins, combined with body movement, are used for moving through the aquatic habitat. In some fish, the fins are modified for a purpose other than movement, such as ensuring egg fertilisation (the fused anal fin is called a *gonopodium*) and protection from predators. The fin positions on the fish body often indicate lifestyle

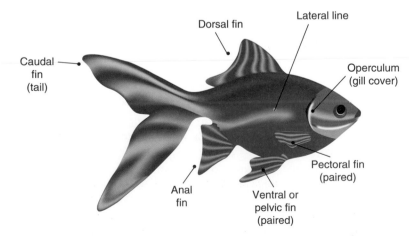

Fig. 17.21   Fish: external fins.

(as predator or prey may need to be capable of continued speed or only short bursts, respectively).

- The position of the mouth may also indicate where that fish feeds, which, in turn, indicates where in the aquarium it will spend most of its time. For example, fish with barbels (feelers) around the mouth parts feed on or near the bottom and others feed and swim in the top layer of the water, whereas fish that live in shoals live and feed in the middle layer of water.
- The eyes vary in size and sight ability, depending on lifestyle. Plant eaters have poor eyesight but a good sense of smell to find food. Predatory fish have good eyesight, enabling them to catch their prey.
- Nostrils, connected to the brain by nerves, provide a sense of smell for food location.
- Gills are located beneath the gill cover (operculum), allowing the fish to extract oxygen from the surrounding water.
- The lateral line is a fluid-filled tube below the skin surface on the sides of the fish, seen as a line of tiny pores opening to the water outside. It is unique to fish and is an organ of hearing. It detects vibrations in the water, alerting the fish to danger, obstacles in its way and food location.

Head types

- The shape of a fish's head can indicate its location in the aquarium.
- Those with an undershot mouth, fringed with barbels, tend to feed on the bottom of the tank.

Internal anatomical features

- The heart has only two chambers.
- The swim bladder, which is filled with gas, helps to maintain buoyancy in the water in most fish.

Tropical freshwater fish

- Tropical freshwater fish have a life span of approximately three years.
- Tropical freshwater fish are found in waters around the world, the temperature of which will vary (21–29°C) depending on altitude, i.e. mountain stream, lake, river pool or sea-level swamp.
- Some fish species in the wild may be found in many continents or only in one lake or river.

Tropical freshwater fish can be divided into two main groups:

- Egg layer, hatching into fry (i.e. gouramis, tetras, barbs)
- Live-bearer, giving birth to fully formed young which are larger than fry (i.e. platies, guppies)

Coldwater fish

- Coldwater fish have a life span of approximately 6–20 years.
- Coldwater fish are found in a range of habitats in the wild. The water temperature (10–23°C), the oxygen levels, the speed of the water current and the water chemistry will vary depending on location, i.e. lakes, ponds, streams and mountain streams.

The two fish commonly kept from this group are:

- Goldfish
- Koi carp

Goldfish

Goldfish varieties are increasingly diverse as a group.
Ideal conditions for a goldfish are:

- Water – neutral pH to slightly alkaline
- Temperature – 10–26°C
- Region – bottom, top and middle

They fall into three main categories:

- Common – the most popular in terms of the number owned; they are a hardy fish, able to live in aquarium or pond
- Single tailed – known for fast swimming ability; the Shubunkin is ideal for a home aquarium, whereas the Comet is better in a pond or large aquarium
- Double tailed – are more unusual and a less hardy type. They are only suitable for deep aquaria and indoor pools. They tend to have a shorter life span due, in part, to their egg-shaped bodies and flotation problems, i.e. Veiltail

Koi carp

Koi originated from Eastern Asia (Caspian and Aral seas) and China. They are ornamental varieties of the common carp and can be very valuable.
Ideal conditions for Koi:

- Water – neutral pH and moderately hard
- Temperature – 10–24°C
- Tank region – top, middle and bottom

Koi are messy feeders, requiring a good filtration system to keep the water clear. They tend to destroy plants; therefore, the furnishings in an aquarium tend to be bogwood or smooth rock. Koi can be mixed with fancy goldfish if required.

Considerations when setting up an aquarium

(1) Size of aquarium
    Standard aquaria can be bought in various combinations of length, width and depth, depending on:
      • The species being kept, e.g. the Veiltail goldfish requires a deeper tank because of the size of its double tail
      • Stocking density of fish to be kept

(2) Positioning of the aquarium
      • Firm foundation – the floor must be able to support the weight of the water-filled tank, ideally over joists not just floor boards
      • Away from draughts, heaters and direct sunlight, i.e. not near a window or in a conservatory
      • In an area of a room that has no passing traffic
      • In a quiet area, too dark for a house plant
      • Next to more than one electrical socket
      • Level the tank and place polystyrene or a foam mat under the tank on the stand to cushion it from any unevenness in the metalwork of the stand

(3) Substrates
    Substrates are materials placed on the bottom of the tank (Fig. 17.22). They include:
      • Coarse gravel – best for large tanks; it is used to recreate the bed of a river or stream
      • Medium and fine gravel – often mixed and can be used with under-gravel filtration
      • Coloured gravel – gaudy but fun; buy from reputable sources to ensure the dyes used are not poisonous
      • Sand – very useful for bottom-dwelling species of fish (there are no sharp points that can injure the fish) and a good substrate for plant growth

Ensure that, whatever the substrate used, it is washed to remove dust particles, dirt and other impurities.

(4) Filtration system
    Filter systems are used to clean the water, filtering out wastes such as excess food materials, sections of plants and fish excretions. A variety of filtration systems are available:
      • External power filters draw water through the various filter media and pump the clean water back into the tank. These are useful for a smaller aquarium set-up
      • Internal power filters also draw water through the various filters but are located inside the tank
      • Under-gravel filters consist of one or more perforated plates that cover the base of the aquarium. An air stone or line is attached to a length of tubing, and the plates are covered by substrate material. The flow of oxygenated water through the gravel allows filtering

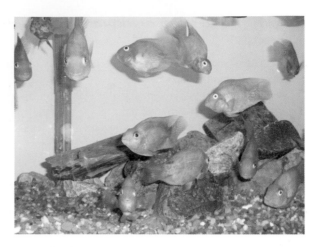

Fig. 17.22   Marine tank substrate.

(a)   (b)

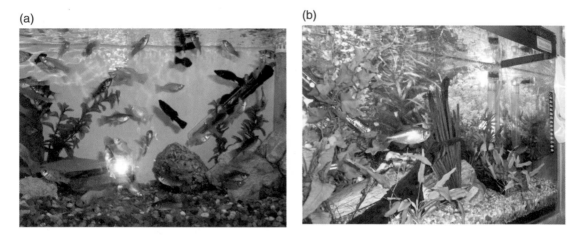

Fig. 17.23   (a) Aquarium heater located in the tank. (b) Fish in an established tank.

(5)   Heating

Heating is used in both coldwater and tropical freshwater tank systems, which require a stable water temperature whatever the environmental temperature may be (even in centrally heated houses, the temperature alters between day and night). Various designs of heater are available (always read the manufacturer's instructions on adjusting the temperature):

- Combined electronic heater/thermostats are located inside the tank (Fig. 17.23)
- Submersible heaters controlled by external or internal thermostats
- Under-tank heating mats controlled by external or internal thermostats

(6)   Aquarium hood or cover

- Prevents dust and dirt particles from falling into the tank
- Prevents fish from escaping

- Keeps out predators such as other household pets
- Helps to retain the tank temperature
- Reduces evaporation

(7) Lighting

Lighting supported in the aquarium hood is essential for the health of the fish and live plants in the tank. Fluorescent tubes have been developed in a number of different colours to imitate daylight and can be used in combination to show off the fish colours.

Setting up the aquarium

- The aquarium tank is cleaned with dilute detergent to remove any chemicals, rinsed thoroughly and put into position.
- In order to hide the electrical cables and filter pipes, choose a decorative plastic background to suit the type of ornament in the tank, the plants and the fish or have a plain black background. This is a personal choice.
- Next, the filter, substrate (gravel or sand), the heater if required, thermometer, prepared wood, rocks and other furnishings are placed.
- Using cold or warm water poured from a clean measuring jug onto a saucer to prevent disturbance of the substrate gravel, begin to fill the tank. Water can be pre-conditioned by allowing it to stand for several days or by adding a conditioner. This allows evaporation of any chlorine gas.
- If the substrate gravel has been washed properly, there should be little or no clouding of the water as it is added. Once the gravel has been covered, water can be poured in quite quickly to about 10–12 cm from the final water level. Plants (plastic) can be placed when the tank has matured, without overflowing.
- It is important to wait at least 24 hours after the set-up has been run before placing any living plants. This allows time to check that the heater and filter are working properly.
- Before the fish can be added, the tank must be at the correct temperature, maturity and pH. Depending on which water company provides the water, it is either:
  - hard: a measure of the mineral salts dissolved in the water
  - soft: indicating fewer dissolved mineral salts
  - acid: pH up to 7
  - alkaline: pH from 7 up to 14
- Coldwater fish are adaptable to a wide range of pH but are most stable in water with a reading of pH between 7 and 8.5. Most tropical freshwater fish will live in water with a pH value between 6.5 and 7.5, which is about neutral in value, and from slightly soft to slightly hard water. There are kits available to check the pH levels.
- Once the tank is set up, it is best for it to be left for at least 3–4 weeks for the filtration system to mature; however, after 10 days the first few fish can be added, waiting a week to introduce the next few. The final number should be in place by 6 weeks, to give a healthy aquarium environment.
- Bacteria will develop in the filter sponge and assist in the breakdown of waste produced by the fish (ammonia is converted to nitrites by bacteria; nitrites are converted to nitrates in the filtration system). To ensure that both fish and live

plants are healthy, maintenance of water quality must take place weekly. A check on the nitrite level using a test kit will indicate whether a partial water change is required.

The nitrogen cycle in an aquarium

- Waste matter from the aquarium plants, uneaten food, faeces and urine from the fish will all contaminate the tank.
- As they decompose, ammonia is formed, which is poisonous to the fish.
- The bacteria in the water break down the ammonia into nitrites and then nitrates, which are harmless to fish and act as a fertilizer for the live plants in the tank. This completes the nitrogen cycle.

Feeding Fish

Types of food:

- Live food (daphnia, brine shrimp and bloodworm)
- Commercial food (freeze dried, tablet, dried flakes, floating food sticks and sinking granules)

The most convenient foods are the commercially produced flake or pellet foods. These provide the correct nutrient requirements and, unlike live foods, are free from the hazards of parasite or disease introduction.

Most coldwater fish kept in aquariums are omnivorous (feeding on insects and plant material). A good-quality flake food will provide the nutrients, vitamins and minerals required, but to keep the fish in good health, alternate this diet with other safe live food, such as daphnia or bloodworm.

Tropical freshwater fish also benefit from variety in their diet. Use of dried flake foods combined with frozen or live foods offered once or twice per week will maintain condition and health. If the fish are herbivorous, offer green foods, such as lettuce leaves, regularly.

Aquarium tank maintenance

Daily

- Check the fish
- Check all the tank equipment
- Make sure that the temperature is correct
- Remove any uneaten food

Every 2 weeks

- Test for pH and nitrite levels
- Do a partial water change

- Remove any dead plant material
- Remove any algal growth from the glass front and sides
- Suction off any debris seen on the sand or gravel substrate

Once a month

- Clean the filter

Every 8–12 months

- Replace fluorescent tube lights and air stones
- Service filter motor and air pump
- Take out and scrub all furniture and plastic plants to remove algae

Reptiles, amphibians and invertebrates

The keeping of reptiles, amphibians and invertebrates as pets has increased greatly over the past decade. Data collected in 2012 indicates that there are approximately 1 million animals from this group kept as pets. The notion of having a pet that is slightly different along with a greater number of hobbyists and also the increase of allergies in children has contributed to this increase in keeping these species groups as pets. Whether or not these species can be classed as pets is debatable as they have not been domesticated in particular and neither are they kept specifically as companions. The keeping of these species of animal as pets could be widely debated.

Keeping reptiles, amphibians and invertebrates brings husbandry demands that can be greater than for any other species with the exception of fish species. Consideration must be given to:

- Dietary needs
- Size of adult animal
- Lighting and heating needs of the species
- Daily management requirements
- Appeal to all household members

Of the animals in this group, reptiles are the most popular – these can be broadly divided into lizards and snakes.

Housing reptiles

Reptiles are housed in accommodation called a *vivarium*. There are many different styles on the market at the current time (2013), and consideration should be given to the needs of the animal intending to be kept in it before choosing the type of vivarium. Buying the cheapest/most expensive vivarium or the one that looks most appealing to the owner may not be the one that suits the needs of the animal.

Consider the following:

- Construction material – wood, plastic, moulded fibreglass and glass are common construction materials for vivaria – all have their advantages and disadvantages.
- Size of the adult animal – be wary of saying that biggest is best for reptiles – some reptiles do not like to have lots of space and so be aware of the species' needs.
- Lifestyle of the animal – an arboreal or burrowing animal will need a taller or deeper enclosure than a ground dwelling one.
- Security of the vivarium – snakes can be experts at escaping from accommodation and so the vivarium should be easily secured to avoid escapes and also avoid other animals or young children from entering the accommodation.
- Provision of life-sustaining systems – heating and lighting – how will these be provided for in the vivarium intending to be chosen?
- Ability to provide the necessary substrate for the species – there are a range of substrates available on the market, and not all of them are suitable for all species of reptile as they can be ingested and cause impaction problems. Substrates are often used for aesthetic appeal to provide a natural-looking environment rather than to meet the needs of the animal. Newspaper is considered by some to be the most suitable substrate (most newspaper inks are now non-toxic).
- Ease of cleaning and maintaining hygienic conditions – there are many furnishings and decorations that can be purchased for the vivaria but consider whether they are needed for aesthetic appeal or for the animal itself. Some furnishings can be provided that make the vivarium more interesting for the animal, e.g. rocks can be provided to hide behind/under or to use for assisting with skin shedding.
- Ease of feeding/water changing – consider the diet of the animal and how it can be met and provided for. Also consider how water should be provided in the vivarium and whether a bowl is needed for bathing or swimming in.
- Access point into the vivarium – just as with mammals, the access points should be at a place where the reptile will not perceive you as a predator.

Heating the vivarium

Heat provision is one of the most important aspects in reptile husbandry as reptiles are unable to maintain their own body temperature. They are *ectothermic* and so rely on the external provision of a heat source to maintain their health and activity levels. A reptile that is too cold will enter a state of torpor and may well appear to have died. Too much heat can cause the animal to become stressed if it cannot move away from the heat source, and this can also result in death or injury.

There are different sources of heat that can be provided in a reptile, and all have their advantages and disadvantages. Spot lamps are popular choices as they can be used to provide a 'basking hotspot' for the animal, but care must be taken to ensure that the animal cannot touch the bulb in any way or that the bulb is securely fixed so as not to fall onto the animal; otherwise, burn injuries could occur. An alternative to spot lamps are ceramic bulbs which emit heat to the surrounding area, but again, the same precautions must be taken. It is also worth noting that the siting of the bulb in the vivarium should not be in a place where the owner/keeper/carer could injure themselves as they can cause serious burns to humans also. Cages can be fitted around bulbs for protection of both animal and owner.

Heat mats/pads are useful as a heat source, but instructions must be carefully followed in order to ensure they have maximum effect without compromising the animal. Heat rocks should not be used as there have been many reported incidences of burn injuries caused to animals.

Within a vivarium, whatever heat source is provided, it is essential to have a *thermal gradient*. This means that the vivarium will be hotter at one end than at the other. This enables the reptile to have a choice of where to be in the enclosure to regulate its body temperature.

A thermostat can be used to regulate the temperature of the heat source provided, and additionally, a timer can be used to replicate the natural temperature cycles in the animal's natural environment.

Humidity in the vivarium

Humidity is an important factor to consider when housing reptiles, and if incorrect, it can affect the health of the animal either by causing cracked skin if too dry for the animal or encouraging fungal infections if too damp. It is essential to research the humidity levels required for the species intending to be kept.

Lighting in the vivarium

Lighting may be provided in a vivarium for a number of reasons, from allowing the animal to be seen to mimicking the light cycles of the natural environment, but the most important reason is to provide ultraviolet rays which aid in the metabolism of calcium. Many captive reptiles suffer from metabolic bone disease due to having incorrect lighting combined with an incorrect diet provided.

When choosing lighting for a vivarium, research how much light the animal intending to be housed requires in terms of strength of light and time required/day. Lights in a vivarium will generally need to be on for 10–12 hours each day.

Light source provision can be controlled through the use of a timer in order to replicate the light cycles of the animal's natural environment.

Light sources should be replaced on a regular basis – every 6 months as a minimum as the strength of a light source diminishes over time.

Hygiene and cleaning in the vivarium

Hygiene is important to both the animal and its owner/keeper/carer. Many reptiles are known to carry the *Salmonella* bacteria which can be transferred to humans as it is zoonotic. High standards of hygiene are therefore vital.

Faeces should be removed on a daily basis. A full clean should be carried out according to the number of animals kept in the vivarium. Substrate should be removed and refreshed on at least a monthly basis. Be wary when using disinfectants with reptiles. It must be ensured that they are suitable for use with reptiles. Seek advice if unsure.

Feeding reptiles

The diet required will depend on the species of animal kept. Many lizards are insectivorous, and this will mean keeping *live food* such as crickets, locusts and mealworm to be fed to the animal. This live food will have specific care requirements in order to keep it alive to feed to the reptile. It is also important to ensure that the live food is provided with a vitamin/mineral supplement on their own food in order to increase the nutritional value of the food to the reptile. Vitamin/mineral deficiencies are common problems in captive reptiles. Advice should be sought on the best supplement to give the species being kept.

Some reptiles are omnivorous and require a small amount of plant matter in their diet, and others are herbivorous and only feed on plant matter. Many reptiles are carnivorous and require vertebrate food.

Invertebrates such as crickets, locusts and mealworms are able to be fed live to those animals that require them. For animals that require small mammals such as mice, rats and gerbils in their diet, it is illegal to feed these animals when they are alive. Any vertebrate food source must be dead when provided to the reptile, and this type of food can be purchased from specialist suppliers and certain pet stores. The feeding habits of the animal being fed should be researched so that the food can be provided in a similar way. With snakes, it is recommended to remove them from their normal accommodation into a separate feeding container, secured with a lid. Snakes should also not be handled for 2–3 days after feeding in order to avoid regurgitating their food which can cause feeding problems subsequently.

Fresh water should be available at all times in a reptile enclosure. The container in which it is provided must be suitable for the species and should be cleaned on a regular basis as the heat and humidity in a vivarium can encourage algal and fungal growth which can be detrimental to the health of the reptile and the owner/carer/keeper. Some species will also defaecate in their water bowl, and this should be cleaned as soon as possible.

Handling reptiles

For many reptiles, handling can be a stressful experience, and so care must be taken to observe the behaviour of the species and recognize signs of stress. Some reptile species will acclimatise more to handling than others. Short, regular sessions of handling will aid this process. During the handling process, it is important to let the animal move freely between hands rather than trying to restrain them in a certain position. Take care with some snakes however as they can coil around parts of the body such as hands, arms, necks etc., in order to secure themselves, and this can constrict the blood flow in the handler. Handling should be a positive experience for both animal and handler.

Section 3
Nursing

Chapter 18
First Aid and Nursing

Summary

In this chapter, the learning outcomes are:

- To identify the aims and objectives of first aid for animals
- To categorise a first aid situation according to its severity
- To describe the initial management of a first aid situation
- To identify the correct method of transporting an injured animal
- To explain the term ABC, describe the recovery position for an animal and describe a body check for an animal
- To describe the life-saving techniques of artificial respiration and cardiac compression for animals
- To describe action to be taken in a range of situations requiring first aid for animals

First aid

First aid is the emergency care and treatment of an animal with sudden illness or injury, before medical and surgical care (veterinary treatment) can be commenced. The main objectives of first aid are to:

- Keep the animal alive
- Make it comfortable
- Assist in pain control
- Prevent its condition getting worse

Different situations where first aid is needed require different approaches. Some situations will allow plenty of time to attend to injuries or problems and never be life threatening. Other situations are so severe that the animal will die if urgent and skilled emergency care is not available.

Animal Biology and Care, Third Edition. Sue Dallas and Emily Jewell.
© 2014 John Wiley & Sons, Ltd. Published 2014 by John Wiley & Sons, Ltd.
Companion Website: www.wiley.com/go/dallas/animal-biology-care

First aid, being only the initial actions of someone attending or witnessing an accident, is very limited. It does not involve diagnosis or medical treatment of injuries, but is designed to preserve life and temporarily prevent a condition getting worse, if possible. It should allow time to get the animal to a veterinary surgeon who can diagnose the full extent of the condition, which is not always obvious at first.

Evaluating situations requiring first aid intervention

Very severe

These are situations which *need immediate action* or the animal will die:

- The heart has stopped (*cardiopulmonary arrest*)
- Breathing is obstructed due to an object in the air passages
- Breathing has stopped
- Bleeding from a main artery or vein
- Acute allergic reaction to insect sting or other substance

Severe

These are situations where first aid action must be taken within one hour or the animal may die:

- Deep cuts and considerable blood loss
- Established shock
- Head injuries
- Breathing difficulties

Serious

These are situations where first aid action must be taken within 4–5 hours or more serious problems will develop that could be life threatening:

- Bone fractures that puncture through the skin (*compound fractures*)
- Spinal injuries
- Early stages of shock
- Difficulties in giving birth (*dystocia*)

Major

In these situations, first aid action must occur within 24 hours to prevent further damage:

- Fractures with no skin injury (*simple fractures*)
- Prolonged vomiting and diarrhoea
- Foreign bodies in the eyes or ears

Initial management of a first aid situation

(1) *Assess the situation and keep calm* – briefly examine the animal and note obvious injuries

(2) *Contact the veterinary practice* – for advice and to let them know you are coming

(3) *Ensure your own safety* – make sure the animal is properly restrained before handling and lifting, so that no one is bitten

(4) *Stop and cover any obvious bleeding* – use sterile dressings if possible to prevent further contamination

(5) *Make sure the animal is able to breathe* – if the airway is obstructed, clear it

(6) *Treat for shock* – by maintaining the body temperature

Handling and transport of an animal requiring first aid

If the animal's life is in danger, then it must be moved. Injured animals are usually in pain, shocked and frightened and may attack anyone who tries to approach or handle them. In order to protect both the handler and the animal from further harm or injury, great care is needed at this time:

- Slow, deliberate movements are essential
- A calm, soothing voice will help
- Handle the animal as little as possible
- Muzzle if necessary and only if the animal has no breathing difficulties
- Transport to the surgery

Before moving the animal, quickly assess the condition. This is referred to as *initial help*, and if this can be started as soon as possible, the chances of survival are greatly improved. The initial assessment and help given must then be reported to the veterinary staff on arrival at the surgery, in order to reduce delay in treatment.

Checks to make are as follows:

- *Airway* – to ensure it is not obstructed; if it is, then clear it if safe to do so
- *Breathing* – to make sure this is possible and assist with artificial respiration if required
- *Circulation – heart and pulse* – check the beat, its rate and strength, and record the information. If the heart has stopped, then proceed with heart massage.

Species consideration is important when considering handling. The method for moving an injured dog will vary from the method used for rodents, horses, cattle or birds, for example.

Transportation of small dogs, cats, rabbits and smaller pets

Transport in a pet carrier or in a cat-sized basket, making sure there are plenty of breathing holes. Many owners now own a cat cage, which is ideal for many species, provided there is plenty of space to stretch out (Fig. 18.1). Alternatively, and depending on the injury, the animal can be held in the owner's arms although this is not recommended (Fig. 18.2).

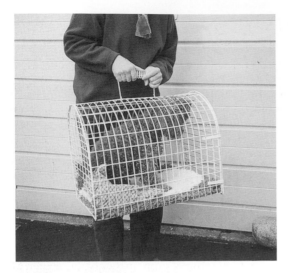

Fig. 18.1 Carrier cage for a small dog or cat.

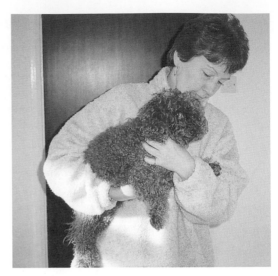

Fig. 18.2 Small dog held in arms.

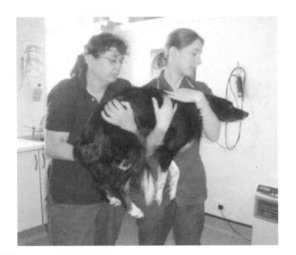

Fig. 18.3 Medium dog lift.

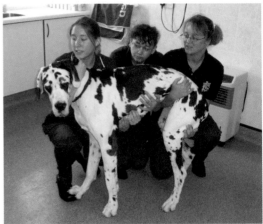

Fig. 18.4 Giant breed lift.

Transportation of medium-sized dogs

If the animal only has minor injuries, then they may be encouraged to walk slowly. If they are not able to walk, then pick them up with one arm around the front of the forelegs and one around the hind legs (providing this is not contraindicated by the injuries), lift and hold against your body, with the legs hanging downwards (Fig. 18.3).

Large breeds of dog or similar

These should only be lifted by more than one person, one supporting the head and chest and another supporting the abdomen and hindquarters (Fig. 18.4). If the dog is too large for lifting, then with two or more handlers, use a stretcher or blanket lift (Fig. 18.5). Pull

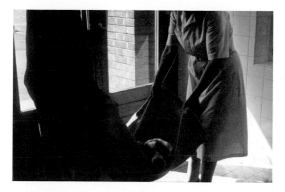

Fig. 18.5 Blanket lift requires two or more people for a large dog.

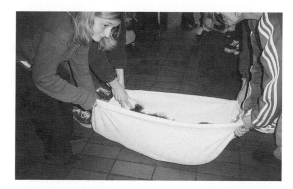

Fig. 18.6 Blanket lift for a smaller dog with spinal injuries.

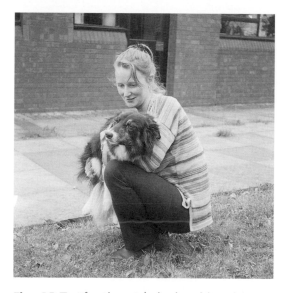

Fig. 18.7 Lift with straight back and bent knees to prevent back strain injury of the handler.

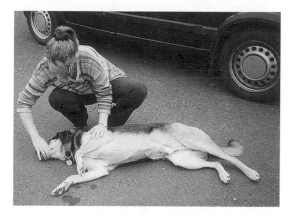

Fig. 18.8 Recovery position for an injured animal, keeping the airway straight.

the animal onto the blanket, lying on its side, and lift using the corners of the blanket or, if not enough handlers are available, simply drag the blanket, provided the surface is smooth. This blanket technique is also used for smaller animals with spinal injuries (Fig. 18.6).

Whatever the size of the injured animal, always lift in the correct manner; bend your knees before lifting rather than bending from the waist (Fig. 18.7). The handler's own back is less at risk, but if in doubt, get more help.

Recovery position for an animal

As in human first aid, in animal first aid, there is a *recovery position* in which to place the animal to ensure breathing is assisted and the heart is exposed for emergency procedures, if required (Fig. 18.8).

- Lie the animal on its right side
- Straighten the head and neck
- The tongue is pulled forwards and behind the canine tooth (to one side of the mouth)
- Remove any collar or harness
- Check the heart and pulse regularly

Other checks to make and record at this time include the following:

- Any signs of *bleeding* from the animal's surface or from a body opening, such as the mouth, rectum, vulva, prepuce or ears.
- *Colour* is checked by looking at the lining of the lower eyelid and the mucous membrane of the mouth and gums. Capillary refill can also be checked when examining the mucous membranes at this time.

Colour of mucous membranes

- *Pale* – indicating shock or serious bleeding (internal or external)
- *Blue* – also referred to as *cyanotic*, indicates lack of oxygen to the tissue cells
- *Yellow* – also referred to as *jaundice*, can be caused by an excess of bile pigment in the bloodstream and usually involves the liver in some way
- *Red/congested* – indicates over-oxygenation after exercise, in heat stroke cases or fever conditions
- The *capillary refill time* is checked. The upper lip is lifted and the gum over the top canine tooth is pressed. This squeezes the blood out of the surface capillaries, causing the area to go temporarily white. The refill time is the time it takes for the gum to become the normal pink colour again as the capillaries refill, usually 1–1½ seconds. Any time longer than that is considered 'slow' and may indicate a degree of shock.
- *Rate and quality of the pulse.* This is taken in the groin area of the hind leg, on the femoral artery. This artery is exposed over the femur bone at this point, allowing the pulse to be taken. Another artery that may be used is the sublingual, under the animal's tongue, but this is only used in unconscious animals. *Rate* refers to the speed of the pulse, which is a reflection of the heartbeat. The pulse should be taken for a full minute for a true recording. The *quality* of the pulse refers to whether it is strong, thready, weak or normal. In order to describe this, the handler must have some experience of pulse taking.
- *Breathing rate* is recorded, describing whether it is normal, slow, fast or shallow.
- *Body temperature* is taken if a thermometer is available. If not, then feel the extremities of the body, such as the feet and tail end. If the temperature is lower than it should be, the handler will feel this, because the normal body temperature of most animals (mammals and birds) is higher than that of humans.
- Record its *level of consciousness*; in other words, can the animal respond to stimuli like its name, a noise or sudden movement?
- Record any *unusual odour* on the animal's body, whether it comes from the animal's mouth, anus or coat.

Life-saving techniques

Life-saving techniques will be needed in two situations that may occur as a result of illness, injury or sudden trauma:

(1)   The heart has stopped – *cardiac arrest*
(2)   The breathing has stopped – *respiratory arrest*

The previously mentioned situations are jointly referred to as *cardiopulmonary arrest* (*pulmonary* refers to the vessels that take blood to the lungs and back to the heart).

The objective of cardiopulmonary resuscitation is to restore heart and lung action and prevent the irreversible brain damage that would happen if the tissues were deprived of oxygen for any length of time. Damage to body cells is thought to occur after 3–4 minutes following cardiac arrest. Therefore, being adequately prepared is the most important step in the management of these emergencies and recognizing that time is short if permanent damage to body tissues is to be avoided.

Cardiac compression (heart massage)

The aim of cardiac compressions is to keep blood moving through the body, thereby providing the oxygen that may be left in the blood to the tissues. The amount of pressure and rate of compressions will depend on the size of the animal.

Small dogs or cats or other small animals

- Place in recovery position (on its right side, head and neck extended and tongue pulled forwards)
- Take hold of its chest between the thumb and fingers of the same hand, over the heart and just behind the elbows
- Support the body of the animal with the other hand on the lumbar spine area
- At all times, keep the head and neck in a straight line to assist breathing
- Squeeze the thumb and fingers of the hand over the heart together; this will compress the chest wall and the heart, which is squeezed between the ribs
- Repeat this action approximately 120 times per minute
- Watch for the heart contractions restarting

Medium-sized dogs and other species

- Place in the recovery position
- Put the heel of one hand on the top of the chest, just behind the elbow and over the heart (Figs. 18.9 and 18.10)
- Place the other hand either on top of the first hand or under the animal to support the heart as it is compressed
- Press down onto the chest with firm, sharp movements
- Repeat this action about 80–100 times per minute
- Watch for the heart contractions restarting

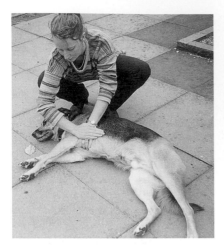

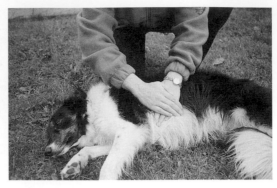

Fig. 18.10 Same hand position, behind the elbow, over the heart.

Fig. 18.9 Position for hands when doing cardiac massage.

Large, barrel-chested or fat dogs and other species

- Place on its back, with its head slightly lower than its body, if possible
- Put the heel of one hand on the abdominal end of the sternum (breast bone)
- Place the other hand on top of the first
- Press firmly onto the chest, pushing the hands forwards towards the head of the animal
- Press down in this way 80–100 times per minute
- Keep the head and neck straight during the procedure, at all times
- Watch for the heart restarting

With all animals, stop at 20 second intervals to check for heartbeat or pulse, and then continue with compressions until further help arrives.

Respiratory arrest

Whatever the cause, if the breathing has stopped, then it must urgently be restarted. Resuscitation methods do include the use of drugs that stimulate the heart and the breathing, but these are only administered by a veterinary surgeon and therefore are not a first aid procedure.

There are two methods for restarting the breathing:

(1) Artificial respiration – manual method
(2) Mouth-to-nose technique

Artificial respiration

- Place in recovery position
- Clear airway of any blocking material

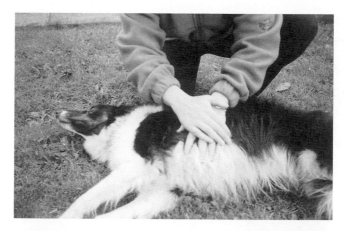

Fig. 18.11   For artificial respiration compression, hands are placed over the chest.

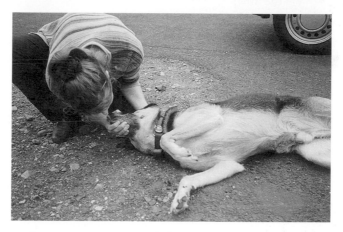

Fig. 18.12   Mouth-to-nose resuscitation with the airway kept straight and mouth held shut. The operator breathes down the nose.

- Place a hand over the ribs, behind the shoulder bone (Fig. 18.11)
- Compress the chest with a sharp, downward movement
- Allow the chest to expand and then repeat the downward movement
- Repeat approximately every 3–5 seconds, until breathing restarts
- Keep head and neck straight at all times to maintain airway

Mouth-to-nose technique

- Place in recovery position
- Clear the airway
- Place a tissue or thin cloth over the animal's nose (for personal safety)
- Hold the animal's neck straight at all times
- Keep its mouth closed by holding upper and lower jaws together
- Breathe down its nose to inflate the lungs (Fig. 18.12)

- Repeat this inflation of the lungs at 3–5 second intervals
- Watch for the breathing restarting

This technique provides the animal with the unused oxygen in the handler's breath and their exhaled carbon dioxide, which helps to stimulate the breathing or gasp reflex in the animal.

Poisons

A poison or toxin is any substance which, on entry to the body in sufficient amounts, has a harmful effect on the individual. Poisons can gain entry to the body by various means:

- By mouth
- Via the lungs
- Absorbed through the skin surface or directly through a cut/wound

Animals can be poisoned by a multitude of potentially toxic substances, many of which are ordinary household products. The source may be poisonous plants or toxic chemicals used or stored near the animal in the kitchen or utility room, where a dog or cat may have its bed. Such poisons would include:

- Pesticides for the garden, such as slug bait and herbicides
- Rodent killers, such as warfarin poison
- Paint and cleaning solutions for brushes
- Disinfectants such as bleach and toilet cleaners
- Drugs such as aspirin, blood pressure tablets and sleeping tablets

Very few poisons produce distinctive signs. Most cause non-specific signs, such as:

- Becoming aggressive, excited or depressed
- Unsteady on its feet
- Salivating, vomiting and/or having diarrhoea
- Abdominal pain and fitting-type episodes
- Pale, with lowered body temperature
- Slow capillary refill time

The owner/carer/keeper knows best what is normal and what is unusual in their animal, so record all reported information and get in touch with the veterinary surgeon as soon as possible for advice on what to do next. If the owner knows the chemical involved and has the container or packet, take that to the veterinary surgeon too. Unless instructed to make the animal sick, do not attempt to do so as this may cause more harm.

Until the veterinary surgeon takes over:

- Place in recovery position
- Support for any breathing problems

- Keep warm to reduce shock
- Record pulse and heart rate
- Comfort and do not leave unattended

Get to the veterinary surgeon as quickly as possible.

Insect stings

Insect stings usually cause more pain than harm. However, it is possible that an animal may have an allergic reaction to the insect venom, or if the sting is near to the airway, any subsequent swelling could obstruct breathing.

If the venom sac is imbedded in the skin, never squeeze it, as this may inject more venom into the animal. Remove carefully if possible, or leave it in place for the veterinary surgeon to remove in the safety of the practice:

- *Wasp stings* are alkaline. Treatment is therefore with an acid solution, such as household vinegar in the form of a pad or compress.
- *Bee stings* are acidic. Treatment is therefore with an alkali such as bicarbonate of soda mixed with water and soaked into a pad or compress.

Treatment for insect stings aims to neutralise the situation. Unless someone has seen it bite or sting, it is not always possible to know which insect is involved. If this is the case, then apply a cold compress or face flannel filled with ice cubes to the area to reduce the swelling and give some pain control.

Bleeding or haemorrhage

Bleeding or *haemorrhage* is the escape of blood from damaged blood vessels and can cause serious problems. Bleeding heavily can decrease the circulating blood volume enough to cause shock. Bleeding that is less heavy may still cause the tissue cells to be deprived of oxygen, which could be permanently damaging. Even small losses of blood can delay wound healing and contribute to development of an infection. Therefore, any loss potentially puts the animal at risk.

Bleeding may be *external* (obviously seen) or *internal* (not always obvious). Internal bleeding should be suspected after incidents such as road traffic accidents, heavy falls or crush injuries, and so, it is important that the following signs are watched for:

- Membrane colour is pale and getting paler
- Behaviour is dull or listless
- Appears thirsty
- The pulse and breathing rate are fast and may appear feeble
- Feet and tail are cold to the touch
- Body temperature is subnormal
- Capillary refill time is slow

If blood loss is severe, then signs include those of blood loss to vital organs, such as the following:

- The animal becomes restless and will not settle
- It has difficulty breathing
- It may have fitting-type episode
- The animal is unable to stand and becomes unconscious

For reporting purposes, the following information is useful to the veterinary surgeon:

- What type of blood vessel is damaged
- Where the injury is on the body
- When the bleeding started
- Whether the bleeding is internal or on the surface
- Treatments carried out so far

What type of blood vessel is damaged?

(1) *Artery* – blood is bright red (oxygenated) in colour and comes out as spurts, which are synchronised with the heartbeat
(2) *Vein* – blood is dark red (deoxygenated) in colour and is a steady flow
(3) *Capillary* – is bright red and seen as a steady ooze

Methods of stopping bleeding

The following methods are only temporary solutions until the veterinary nurse/surgeon takes over:

Digital (finger) pressure

Use on surface wounds by pressing a sterile or clean pad of absorbent material onto the area to control the blood loss. Care must be used with this method in case there is a foreign body such as metal, glass or material fibres in the wound as pressing directly on this could push it deeper, where it would be harder to locate or may cause damage to internal structures. The direct pressure method could be adapted to aim to press either side of the foreign body if possible.

This method can be used for about 5–15 minutes before tissues beyond must receive a reviving flow. Then pressure can be re-established.

Pressure points

In several locations around the body, major arteries travel near to the body surface. These tend to supply the extremities such as limbs and tail. Where they cross a bone, pressure can slow, or even stop, the supply reaching an area beyond. If the wound is on the extremity, these points can be used as a temporary measure:

- *Forelimbs* – the pressure is put on the inside or medial elbow area, to slow the *brachial artery* flow

- *Hindlimbs* – the pressure is put on the same site used for pulse taking, in the groin area on the femur, to slow the *femoral artery* flow
- *Tail* – the pressure is applied to the ventral or underside of the base of the tail, to slow the *coccygeal artery* flow

These locations can be used for about 5–10 minutes, before allowing the blood to flow to restore distant tissues.

Pressure bandages

These may be used initially or after one or both of the aforementioned methods have been used to establish the extent of the injury.

Pressure bandages can only be applied to extremities, such as limbs and tail. They are applied tightly to constrict and slow the surface vessels supplying the area, thus limiting blood loss.

Plenty of padding material is applied over the dressing on the wound and is then tightly bandaged in place. If blood seeps through, then more padding is applied and bandaged in place.

This is still only a temporary measure to be used before arriving at the veterinary surgery and will give about 1 hour of time before the tissues must be released from the tight bandage and flow restored.

Shock

Shock is a term used to describe a very complex and potentially fatal clinical syndrome which always involves insufficient blood to the tissues, resulting in lack of oxygen to the cells. Lack of oxygen to the cells is called *tissue hypoxia*, and this can be fatal if not corrected.

When blood is lost from the body, the body tries to compensate by redistributing blood to vital structures like the brain and heart, at the expense of other organs like kidneys, skin, intestines and muscles. Organs can be severely damaged by the resulting tissue hypoxia.

The causes of shock vary, but some examples are:

- Blood loss from damaged vessels
- Trauma injuries to tissues from a road traffic accident
- Pain due to injury or surgical procedures
- Heart problems that interfere with its normal pumping action
- Infections that cause blood to 'pool out' in the capillary beds, by affecting the walls of the blood vessels

The *signs of shock* include:

- Pale colour (Fig. 18.13)
- Cold extremities
- Weak or slipping into an unconscious state

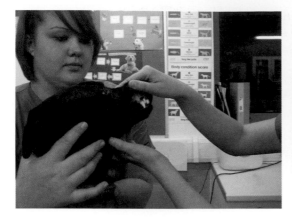
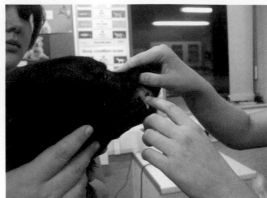

Fig. 18.13 Mucous membrane colour check.   **Fig. 18.14** Capillary refill time check.

- Increase in the heart rate and breathing
- Slow capillary refill time of longer than two seconds (Fig. 18.14)

Until the animal can be treated by a veterinary surgeon, the handler must start the preventive shock procedure. Maintaining body temperature is probably the single most useful thing that can be done. If the body is not allowed to shut down the peripheral vessels to the limbs and tail, shock will be at least delayed and possibly even prevented.

Shock takes three forms:

- *Impending* – it is expected to happen, bearing in mind the events or injuries
- *Established* – it is in place and the animal must have urgent medical treatment involving whole-blood transfusions or use of plasma expanders
- *Irreversible* – treatment is unlikely to save the animal's life as systems are too damaged

Treatment is aimed at not allowing shock to move beyond the impending stage. To achieve this:

- Maintain body temperature by wrapping in blankets or towels (Fig. 18.15) and keep massaging or rubbing the extremities to stimulate the blood flow. Never use artificial heat as the temperature may get too high
- Position the head slightly lower than the body to encourage the blood flow to the brain
- Stop any further blood loss
- Assist the animal to breathe by placing in the recovery position, and give artificial respiration if breathing stops
- Record the pulse
- Get to the veterinary surgery as quickly as possible

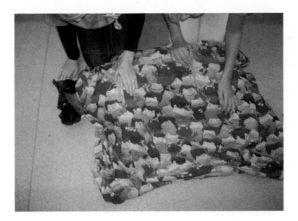

Fig. 18.15 Maintaining body temperature.

Heat stroke (hyperthermia)

Heat stroke results from an excessive rise in body temperature caused by high environmental temperatures. Dogs and cats do not lose body temperature through the skin due to their dense coats and lack of sweat glands. Therefore, to eliminate excess body heat, they use the respiratory system, inhaling cool air through the nose and exhaling hot air from the body through the mouth. The faster this exchange occurs, the faster their body will cool down, which is why dogs pant after exercise. Heat stroke is rarely seen in cats, and in dogs, it usually occurs because the animal has been confined, on a hot day, with no access to shade, or in a car/vehicle with insufficient ventilation.

NB: On a hot day, the temperature in a car soon becomes higher than the environmental temperature, even if windows are left open. **Do not leave dogs in cars on a hot day** even if parked in the 'shade'.

When the environmental temperature exceeds the animal's body temperature, it ultimately becomes impossible to maintain body temperature within normal limits for that animal.

Heat stroke affects all dogs, but those most at risk, if exposed to excess heat, are:

- Those with thick dense coats
- Overweight animals
- Short-nosed breeds
- Animals with heart conditions
- Elderly animals
- Animals with medical conditions that affect the breathing

Panting becomes ineffective and the body temperature will rise rapidly; death follows quickly if the body temperature is not immediately reduced.

Signs of heat stroke include:

- Excess panting and salivation
- Bright red mucous membranes (check the gums)
- Vomiting
- Excitement/anxiety
- Disoriented
- Collapsed/unable to stand
- Body temperature high (41–43°C)

It is essential to reduce body temperature urgently:

- Remove the animal from the hot environment
- Cool the animal using:
  o a pack of frozen vegetables held on the neck area
  o wrap in towel/blanket soaked with cold water, and continue to hose water over the soaked wrapping, keeping clear of the face
- Monitor the animal's body temperature
- If collapsed, put into the recovery position to assist breathing
- If conscious, encourage to drink restricted amounts of water continuously (if unrestricted, the animal may swallow too much water too quickly and cause vomiting)
- Treat for shock if the temperature falls below normal

Hypothermia

Hypothermia is commonly seen in young or small animals, due to an inability to control body temperature within normal limits. This may be caused by illness or accident, leaving the animal unable to restore temperature loss unless assisted.

Signs of hypothermia include:

- The animal appears sleepy or lethargic
- Its movement becomes weaker
- It is unconscious

Treatment of hypothermia includes:

- If the animal is wet, dry it by rubbing vigorously with a towel
- Wrap, using a lightweight covering, to preserve heat
- Increase the environmental temperature but do not overheat
- Monitor constantly by taking temperature and do not leave unattended

Bone fractures

A fracture refers to an incomplete or complete break in a bone's structure. Breaks in the bone are usually obvious but may not always be, and so, the objectives of first aid for fractures are to prevent the situation from getting worse and make the animal comfortable for transportation to the veterinary surgery.

The causes of bone fracture are varied and include:

* Road traffic accidents
* The animal landing badly after jumping
* Muscles contracting to break small bones, particularly in the legs of racing dogs or horses
* Bone disease that has weakened the bone structure

Types of fracture

Fractures are classified according to the type of break and associated damage:

* *Simple* – the bone is completely broken but there is no connecting skin injury (Fig. 18.16)
* *Compound* – the bone is completely broken, and there is a wound connecting to the skin, or the bone is protruding through the skin. A badly handled simple fracture can become a compound fracture
* *Greenstick* – the break in the bone is incomplete. This type of break is often seen in young animals as their bones are softer than adult animals and so appear to bend like a young twig on a tree

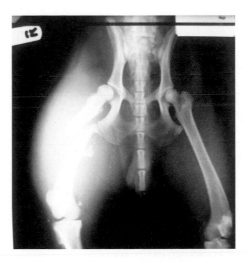

Fig. 18.16 X-ray shows fractured right femur and extent of tissue swelling.

The signs indicating a fracture include:

- Loss of use of the affected limb (animal will not bear weight)
- Pain on handling or will not allow handling
- Unusual position or shape to the limb – usually obvious to see
- Swelling and bruising
- Unusual movement of the limb

The best treatment for fractured bones is to get the animal to the veterinary surgery quickly, but taking care to cause no further injuries by careless handling. Some fractures are also complicated by damage to surrounding tissues, such as blood vessels, nerves or organs.

Depending on the type of fracture, first aid aims to:

- Stop any bleeding.
- Clean and cover any wounds.
- Immobilise the fracture site. This is only possible if the joints above and below the site can be immobilised by a splint. If splinting is possible, always apply the splint to the limb in the position in which it is found. For example, if the foot and carpals of the foreleg are now positioned sideways instead of facing front, do not correct the position – splint it.

The materials that can be used for splinting include:

(1) Rolled-up magazine or newspaper
(2) A ruler or piece of wood
(3) Cardboard
(4) A matchstick

If a splint is not possible, then:

- Confine on plenty of bedding
- Comfort and do not leave unattended
- Treat for shock

What can be splinted?

- *Forelimb* – from elbow to toes (*phalanges*)
- *Hindlimb* – from stifle to toes
- *Tail*

Get to the veterinary surgery as quickly as possible.

Wounds

A wound is damage to the continuous structure of any tissue in the body. The healing process consists of a number of stages until it is complete.

Stages of wound healing

First-intention healing

- This takes place in wounds that:
  - Are not contaminated with grit, soil or micro-organisms
  - Have clean-cut edges that can be held together
  - Have been cleaned within one hour of injury
- In this type of healing, the edges rejoin by 10 days after injury.

Second-intention healing or granulation

- This takes place in wounds that
  - Are contaminated with grit, soil and micro-organisms
  - Have jagged edges and possibly sections of skin missing
  - Have not been cleaned within two hours of injury
  - Have edges that gape open
  - Become infected
- This type of healing can take weeks to months.

Types of wound

Wounds are described as being open or closed.

Closed wounds do not penetrate the whole thickness of the skin as a structure, such as bruises or blood blisters (*haematoma*), or pockets of blood from a small damaged blood vessel. Treatment involves the use of a cold compress, such as ice cubes held in a face flannel, immediately after injury, to reduce the swelling of local tissues and help control pain. This treatment is only useful immediately after injury.

Open wounds are those where damage to surface tissue is also sustained and some bleeding occurs. They are named according to the manner of the damage and whether or not tissue is missing:

(1) *Incised* – these have clean-cut edges and are particularly painful due to surface nerve ending damage and tend to bleed freely. Caused by sharp-edged materials such as glass, metal or knife blade.

(2) *Lacerated* – these have very jagged flaps of skin and sometimes skin sections are missing (*avulsed*). However, because tissue is torn and stretched, they are less painful than incised wounds and do not bleed much. Caused by bite injuries, barbed wire or road traffic accident.

(3) *Puncture* – these wounds have a long, narrow track deep into the tissues, with only a small skin entry scab over the track. The scab holds any microbes in the track. The wound is caused by sharp, pointed objects, such as teeth in bite wounds, nails and thorns. These will all be contaminated with microbes, which are then left in the damage track to multiply, causing a local infection to develop. This local infection

is held in the track area and, as it increases in size, is called an *abscess*. These are very painful, often causing loss of limb function.

(4) *Abrasions* – these have torn, ragged skin edges, with many contaminants embedded in the damaged areas. They are caused by a glancing blow or by being dragged along the ground briefly in a road traffic accident. The tissues tend to be torn and the damage only in the surface layers of the skin, so there is not much bleeding.

Wound care

The sooner an open wound is cleaned using a water-based antiseptic solution, the more chance there is that infection will not develop. The solutions used for wound cleaning must not cause any further inflammation or damage to the wound and therefore should not contain any detergent.

If micro-organisms in the wound are prevented from multiplying, it could mean the difference between the wound healing within 10 days (*first intention*) and the delayed healing of the second-intention or granulation method.

The solutions to use for cleaning a wound include:

- Tap water
- 0.9% sodium chloride from a drip bag
- Antiseptic such as Hibiscrub

Once cleaned, always cover the wound to prevent contamination and further aggravation of the area by the animal.

Eye injuries

Any animal with an eye injury will be sight impaired and in pain, and this will cause substantial changes in the animal's behaviour. It is very important to approach slowly and talk to the animal so that it is warned of your approach. The animal will be frightened and could injure the handler unless precautions are observed and correct handling techniques used (Fig. 18.17).

The types of eye injury that may be seen include the following:

Chemicals

These can cause serious injury to the eye structures. Always irrigate (wash out) as soon as possible, using tap water to remove any chemical. Do not leave the animal unattended and seek medical help immediately.

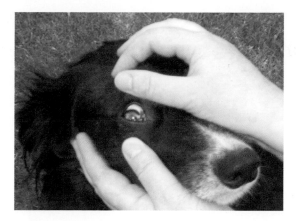

Fig. 18.17   Examine the eye carefully, touching the lids only.

Prolapsed eyeball

This means the eye is now in front of the lids and the optic nerve cord is being stretched as the lids swell. Never touch the eyeball. Treatment is as follows:

- Keep the eye moist at all costs. Use tap water soaked into a pad, squeeze out and apply to the eye area
- Once moistened, soak the pad again in tap water and place gently over the eye
- Hold or bandage in position
- Do not leave unattended and stop any self-mutilation
- Keep warm, quiet and comfortable
- Seek veterinary assistance urgently

The important point to remember is that the eye must not be allowed to dry out. Some breeds of dog, such as Pugs, Pekingese and Boxers, are prone to eye prolapse due to their shortened faces; therefore, always use extra care when handling these breeds.

If the handler is present when the prolapse happens, return the eye by holding the upper and lower eyelids and pulling them gently over the eyeball. This is only possible immediately after injury; do not attempt to do this if the eye has been prolapsed for longer than ten minutes.

Seek assistance from a veterinary surgeon immediately.

Perforating injury

This is usually seen when a sharp instrument becomes embedded in the structure of the eye. Never pull the foreign body out of the eye, even if it is large enough to grasp. If it is removed non-surgically, the front chamber of the eye would leak fluid (*aqueous humour*), causing the back chamber to prolapse forwards, thereby destroying the eye structure.

Treatment is to keep the eye moist, prevent self-mutilation and get to the veterinary surgery quickly.

Chapter 19

Basic Bandaging

Summary

In this chapter, the learning outcomes are:

- To identify the reasons for bandaging to occur
- To identify the aims of bandaging
- To describe how to apply a bandage
- To describe the precautions that should be observed when bandaging an animal

Bandaging is one of the most important skills that can be learnt by an owner/keeper/carer of an animal in order that they can monitor a bandage that has been after injury or surgery.

Reasons for bandaging

- Protect a wound.
- Prevent self-mutilation and interference.
- Support soft tissues (muscle or ligament) in sprains and strains.
- Stop bleeding (pressure bandage).
- Prevent contamination.
- Reduce swelling (cold bandage or pack).
- Hold a dressing in place.

A clinically applied bandage has several different layers for maximum effect. Layers of a bandage are:

Primary or contact layer

- Dressings are placed on the surface of the skin against the wound to assist healing. The type of dressing is dependent on the type of wound:
  - *Adherent* dressings, i.e. gauze swab, tend to stick to the wound and may be difficult to remove without damaging a layer of new tissue.

Animal Biology and Care, Third Edition. Sue Dallas and Emily Jewell.
© 2014 John Wiley & Sons, Ltd. Published 2014 by John Wiley & Sons, Ltd.
Companion Website: www.wiley.com/go/dallas/animal-biology-care

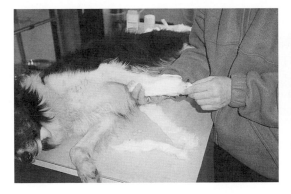

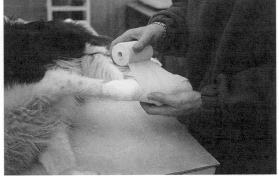

Fig. 19.1 The area to be bandaged is protected with a padding material, between the toes and dewclaw.

Fig. 19.2 A protective layer covers the bandage.

o *Non-adherent* dressings, i.e. Melolin or Rondo, absorb wound fluids into the cotton wool-type backing. They do not stick to wounds or cause so much damage on removal.
o *Moist* dressings, i.e. intrasite, encourage healing.
o Impregnated dressings, e.g. silver or iodine based, to promote rapid healing.

Secondary layer

- This provides the absorption and padding which promotes comfort for the animal.
- Cotton wool (Fig. 19.1), foam and synthetic padding are all suitable materials to use as the secondary layer.

Top layer

- The top layer is known as the conforming layer.
- The top layer secures the primary and secondary layers and protects from the environment and the patient. This is either an adhesive or a self-adherent material, i.e. Elastoplast or Vetrap (Fig. 19.2).
- Examples include open weave bandages, tubular bandages, conforming bandages and crepe bandages (although crepe bandages are now not commonly used).

Aims of bandaging

The bandage must be comfortable. If applied too tightly, the animal will try to remove the bandage or the surface tissues will be damaged by the animal's constant licking.

The aims of bandaging are to:

- Prevent the animal interfering with the area affected under the bandage.
- Limit movement in the case of broken bones or tissue damage and therefore limit pain.
- Stay on for the required amount of time.
- Look neat but will do the job until professional help is reached.

Once the bandage has been applied, then it is necessary to watch out for any of the following:

- Smells coming from the bandage
- Obvious discharge or wound leakage
- Discomfort
- Interference or self-mutilation to try and remove the bandage
- Over-exercising
- Bandage getting wet or dirty
- Any signs of ill health

If any of the signs listed previously are seen in an animal with a bandage, seek advice from a veterinary surgeon straight away.

Rules for bandaging

- Wash hands before starting to prevent introducing infection.
- Get all the materials together before restraining the animal.
- Never stick adhesive tapes onto the animal's coat or hair as it is hard to remove.
- Do not use safety pins or elastic bands to secure the ends of any bandage. Use narrow adhesive tape on the bandage surface.
- In the case of a leg bandage, include the foot; otherwise, it will swell.
- Have the animal restrained in the correct position for application of the bandage.
- If unsure of temperament, always muzzle for safety.

Figures 19.3, 19.4, 19.5, 19.6, 19.7, and 19.8 demonstrate bandaging technique.

Application

It is important to apply the bandage material in a spiral fashion to prevent the development of pressure rings on the skin. When bandaging a limb, it is important to bandage distal to proximal using a figure of eight-spiral pattern. If the bandage is applied in a circular manner, then a *pressure ring* occurs. This can also happen if the bandage is not applied firmly enough and it slips from its original position on the limb to lie as rings over one area.

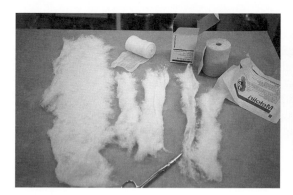

Fig. 19.3 Prepare all materials prior to restraint of the animal.

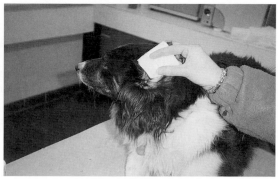

Fig. 19.4 Ear bandage. First, protect the wound with a dressing.

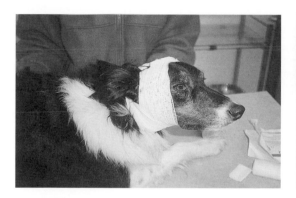

Fig. 19.5 Hold dressing in place with injured ear flap bandaged against the top of the head.

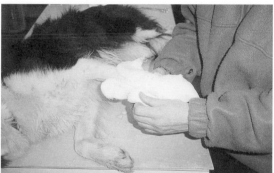

Fig. 19.6 The padding.

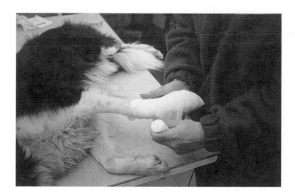

Fig. 19.7 The bandage.

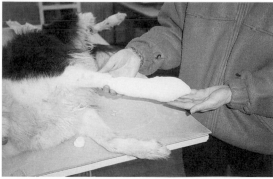

Fig. 19.8 The top protective layer.

A tight bandage can cause fluid to build up in the tissues and prevent its proper flow. To make sure a bandage is not applied too tightly, it should be possible to easily slip two fingers under the edge of the bandage. On limb bandages, only the tips of the toes should be left visible. If exercising an animal outside with a bandaged limb, then several products are commercially available to prevent the bandage from being soiled, e.g. booties. If an animal is paying too much attention to the bandaged area, then initially check that the bandage is suitably applied and use distraction techniques with treats or toys before considering the use of a bitter-tasting spray or an Elizabethan collar to prevent access to the area.

Chapter 20
The Hospital Environment

Summary

In this chapter, the learning outcomes are:

- To identify reasons that an animal may be hospitalised
- To be able to describe the hospital environment for animals
- To describe how a hospitalised animal should be monitored
- To describe the importance of hygiene and cleaning processes in an animal hospital

There are several reasons why animals may be hospitalised:

- Observation
- Operation
- Treatment
- Collection of samples or to run diagnostic tests
- Nursing care

To ensure a high standard of care, there must be adequate facilities, equipment and trained human resources. Locations within the practice for the care of patients include:

- Preparation room
- Preparation/triage room
- Kennels
- Intensive care areas
- Theatre
- Recovery area

Animal Biology and Care, Third Edition. Sue Dallas and Emily Jewell.
© 2014 John Wiley & Sons, Ltd. Published 2014 by John Wiley & Sons, Ltd.
Companion Website: www.wiley.com/go/dallas/animal-biology-care

Environmental temperature in the hospital environment

Most mammals and birds are able to regulate their body temperature to maintain optimum levels. The ideal temperature range varies between species to allow for the working of the internal environment of each, known as *homeostasis*.

The monitoring of body temperature for cold-blooded species such as snakes and lizards is not useful, because they are dependent on the environmental temperature for body function, and so in the hospital environment, a suitable, external heat source must be provided.

In the case of warm-blooded patients who control their own body temperature, help is sometimes needed, however. When conscious and healthy, control is generally good, but when ill or injured, patients may need help from the nursing environment.

Conditions that can cause a raised body temperature are:

- Heat stroke
- Infection
- Stress
- Exercise
- Poisons

Conditions causing a lowered body temperature are:

- Very young/old
- Serious haemorrhage
- Shock
- Recovery from anaesthesia
- Poisons

Patients in the veterinary hospital will benefit, often dramatically, if the environmental temperature is raised or lowered to suit their special needs when, for a variety of reasons, they are unable to maintain it within normal limits themselves.

Methods to assist these patients include:

- Heat pads
- Bubble wrap
- Water-circulating pads
- Incubator
- Hot-water bottles – well wrapped
- Lightweight blankets
- Space blankets
- Vet beds
- Bean bags

Whatever the normal body temperature for the species that is hospitalised, maintain it!

Hygiene and cleaning

The hospital environment will house high concentrations of micro-organisms which are potentially *pathogenic* (can cause disease) to patients. Injured or diseased patients are at risk because of decreased resistance to infection. Every effort must be made to decrease the microbe population in the hospital environment in order to safeguard patients.

In order to protect the patient:

- Eliminate or control the source of the disease – disinfectant and antiseptic use.
- Increase the patient's resistance to disease – e.g. through vaccination and improved diet.
- Prevent the transmission of disease – ventilation, isolation of suspect animals and use of disposable protective clothing.

If mops are used for washing the floor (Fig. 20.1), the following rules should be followed:

- Mop heads should be washed in the washing machine and dried daily.
- If used more than once daily, soak for 30 minutes in a bucket of disinfectant.
- Never leave in soaking solution for more than 30 minutes.
- Wring out thoroughly before use on the floors.

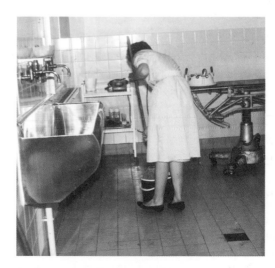

Fig. 20.1   Cleaning the floor area in the theatre.

In use, the mop should be moved from left to right across the body; never pushed back and forwards in front of the operator. Agitate in the disinfectant solution, wring out and proceed to clean. When the area around the operator has been cleaned, then move, repeating the mop rinsing. Start with the area farthest from the door and do not allow anyone to walk on the floor until it is dry.

Change the disinfectant solution between rooms or more frequently if heavily soiled. Use a separate mop and cleaning equipment in the sterile areas such as the theatre suite.

Routine room cleaning

- Remove waste from all bins and replace plastic liner.
- Clean and disinfect walls.
- Spot clean surfaces, cupboard doors, doors, light fixtures, drip stands and any other items routinely kept in this area.
- Check and restock any disposable equipment.
- Clean and disinfect the sinks.
- Clean and disinfect the floor.
- Disinfect and store cleaning equipment.

Different hospital areas require different approaches. The following areas are important:

- Consultation rooms
- Kennels/recovery area
- Triage
- Theatre

Consultation rooms (Fig. 20.2)

- Clean and disinfect all floors and surfaces at the end of the consultation periods (morning, afternoon and evening).
- Collect used instruments, wash and leave ready for sterilizing (if appropriate).
- Dispose of all waste using the correct disposal bags (yellow for clinical waste).
- Use disposable cloth or paper towel only.
- Disinfect all surfaces.
- Empty bins.

Kennels/recovery area (Fig. 20.3)

This area includes the room maintenance and the cage/kennel maintenance. Room maintenance is as for routine cleaning instructions to be carried out at a time which would cause the least disturbance to inpatients as possible. This may be early in the morning before surgery begins or overnight if the hospital has night shift staff.

If an animal is recovering from the procedures, disturb as little as possible, but if soiled, clean out and make comfortable straight away.

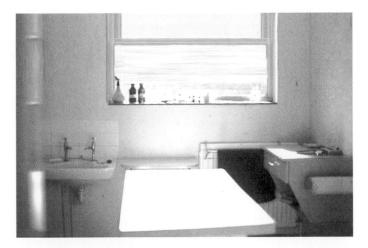

Fig. 20.2   Consultation room.

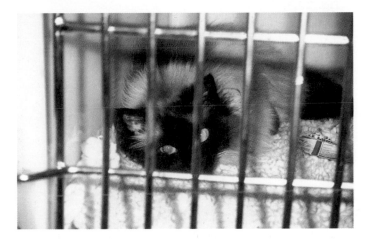

Fig. 20.3   Recovery cage.

Check before disposal of waste materials that a sample is not required (the cage/kennel should be numbered or carry a cage/kennel card) (Fig. 20.4). If a sample is requested by the veterinary surgeon in charge of the case, collect into appropriate container, seal and refrigerate. Make a note on the case card that collection has taken place.

NB: Before any cleaning or collection of samples, put on protective clothing!

Triage area (Fig. 20.5)

Triage refers to the examination and rapid classification of a case. This is one of the most important areas in a modern veterinary hospital. It is here that animals are:

- Examined as inpatients
- Prepared for minor procedures
- Prepared for surgery

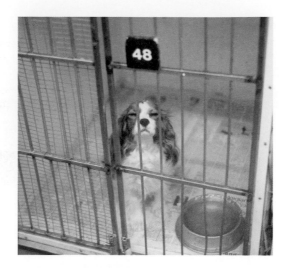

Fig. 20.4 Numbering of kennels for ID purposes.

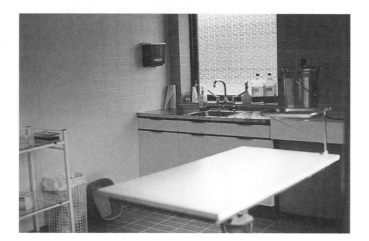

Fig. 20.5 Triage area.

This is a non-sterile area, but because of the variety of patients who pass through this room, it is essential to maintain a high level of hygiene. There will usually be piped oxygen or a mobile oxygen delivery cylinder, plus the emergency treatment drugs and materials for first aid. Pre-operation preparation may include anaesthetising and clipping the site of surgery in triage, which means no cross-contamination of patients takes place as a result of the maintenance of high standards.

To achieve these standards, routine room care includes the following:

- Frequent emptying of all bins and waste collection.
- Collect and/or vacuum up all coat clippings.

- Clean the clippers after each patient and lubricate.
- Spot check and clean the examination tables between patients.
- Dispose of collected urine if, for the purpose of surgery, the animal's bladder has been emptied.
- Check all surfaces and spot clean and disinfect between patients.
- Take any samples for analysis to laboratory or to the office for posting to a distant laboratory.
- Restock supplies.
- Regularly empty the vacuum cleaner and change the bag/filter.
- Clean and disinfect the sink area.

This area is always situated near to the theatre for the easy movement of patients. Also nearby are the areas for:

- Surgical team to scrub up prior to operating
- Sterilising of equipment and instruments
- Packing and cleaning of surgical instruments

These work areas need very high levels of sterility and hygiene. As many procedures take place in this area, it is essential that the order and organisation of equipment are well established. If not, then it is hard for the staff to locate and prepare materials for the necessary procedures.

Systems include:

- Good shelving
- Cupboards and cabinets with obvious labels concerning equipment and use
- Sterilising dates on all packs
- Stock required and location for use

Theatre

Surgery should be conducted in an environment which minimises the chances of introducing micro-organisms into a wound or surgical site. Many micro-organisms commonly associated with people, animals and the environment are potentially pathogenic (disease causing) and can cause wound breakdown and infections.

A surgical wound can be infected from:

- The surgical/theatre environment
- The surgeon and/or surgical team
- The instruments or other equipment
- The patient's own resident micro-organisms which are either internal or external

The modern surgical ritual is designed to address each of these potential sources of infection.

There is a mixture of personnel in this area:

- Those that are scrubbed up and part of the operating team and who may only touch the sterile operating site.
- Those of the non-sterile team who have various duties to perform but are not involved with the surgical areas. They will operate the monitoring systems and maintain anaesthetics and other equipment which supports the surgical procedure.

Personal hygiene for the non-scrubbed team is important although not to the same high standard as the operating team. Non-scrubbed staff have the jobs of:

- Producing equipment required, at the appropriate time
- Tidying away equipment
- Preparing for the next operation

There should be minimal traffic through the theatre because movement increases the distribution of micro-organisms in the atmosphere and therefore could increase the incidence of wound infections. There should be a ventilation system which replaces theatre air with clean air approximately ten times per hour in order to prevent airborne contamination.

On completion of the day's surgical procedures:

- Collect used instruments and place in cold water/detergent solutions ready for cleaning (Fig. 20.6)
- Collect and dispose of all waste
- Spot check and clean all surfaces with disinfectant
- Restock disposable equipment
- Check all other supplies and equipment
- Wipe down walls, operating table and doors with disinfectant

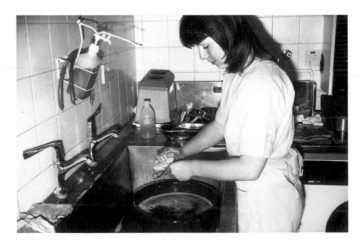

Fig. 20.6 Instruments in cold water/detergent ready for cleaning.

- Vacuum the floor for any hair/coat material
- Mop the floor, starting farthest from the exit door and working towards it
- Ventilate the room
- Before the next operation, 'wet dust' all surfaces with antiseptic solution

Hygiene terms reminder:

- *Sterilisation* – the removal or destruction of all living micro-organisms including bacterial spores.
- *Disinfectants* – will kill pathogenic micro-organisms.
- *Antiseptics* – prevent micro-organism from multiplying and therefore infection fails to develop.
- *Asepsis* – is a state of being free from micro-organisms.

See Chapter 13 for further details relating to hygiene.

Chapter 21
The Hospitalised Patient

Summary

In this chapter, the learning outcomes are:

- To be able to describe husbandry processes relating to the hospitalised patient
- To describe a nursing care plan
- To name examples of nursing models
- To describe the importance of isolation and barrier nursing
- To explain the concept of pathogenic resistance

Any patient that is hospitalised required the utmost care to aid and promote recovery.

Records and monitoring

Records contain owner/pet details and other information which is vital to the veterinary surgeon who must assess the patient's progress (Fig. 21.1):

- Temperature, pulse and respiration rates taken as often as necessary
- Detail on appetite and feeding
- Urine/faeces passed
- Any vomiting episodes

Observation

The veterinary surgeon will examine at least twice daily to assess progress. The nursing staff are responsible for the animal's cleanliness, feeding, watering, medication at correct times and reports on any changes to its condition. The contact time due to the duties discussed earlier allows the nursing staff to:

Animal Biology and Care, Third Edition. Sue Dallas and Emily Jewell.
© 2014 John Wiley & Sons, Ltd. Published 2014 by John Wiley & Sons, Ltd.
Companion Website: www.wiley.com/go/dallas/animal-biology-care

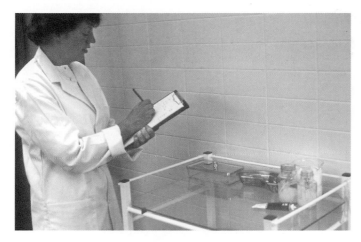

Fig. 21.1 Recording information on patients.

- Observe the patient
- Notice any behavioural changes
- Note the quantity of food eaten and which is its favourite food
- Give detail on whether the faeces is formed or diarrhoeal
- Note if the animal coughs after waking up
- Note whether the animal shows signs of pain or discomfort

Feeding and watering

The cage or kennel should contain a support for feed and water bowls to prevent them from being tipped over. Bowls are always washed and disinfected daily. Fresh water is always available unless prohibited by the veterinary surgeon in charge of the case. A sign is then placed on the front of the housing indicating the patient should not be fed (Fig. 21.2).

Some patients may require measured amounts of water, so that water input and output can be recorded (Fig. 21.3).

Feeding varies with patients but is normally twice daily, as per the hospital routine:

- In the morning to determine the appetite
- In order to assist in the administration of some medicines
- In the case of medical diabetes mellitus, where medicines and food must be timed and regulated
- Postoperatively, patients may need to be encouraged to feed (Fig. 21.4)

Feeding may also be affected for a number of reasons:

- Scheduled for surgery and must have an empty stomach
- Medical condition

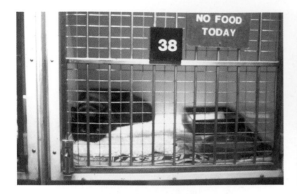

Fig. 21.2 Identify kennels where restrictions are instructed by the attending veterinary surgeon.

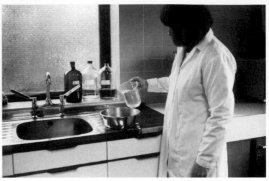

Fig. 21.3 Measure the required amount and record on the record chart.

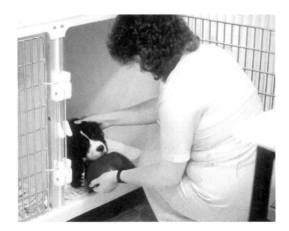

Fig. 21.4 Postoperatively, patients will need to be encouraged to feed.

- After surgery to the gastrointestinal tract
- Requires blood tests
- Is vomiting and/or has diarrhoea

Hygiene

Regular checks are made through the day to make sure no animal lies in a body discharge (Fig. 21.5). After moving the animal from a soiled housing or kennel, check to see if samples need to be collected for investigations.

Mark the cage details, with collection times, then clean and disinfect. To prevent animals from getting soiled, grills may be covered with a layer of bedding to allow a soakaway effect for use with incontinence pads.

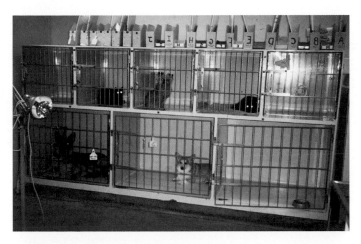

Fig. 21.5   Hospital holding kennels allow easy monitoring for signs of soiling.

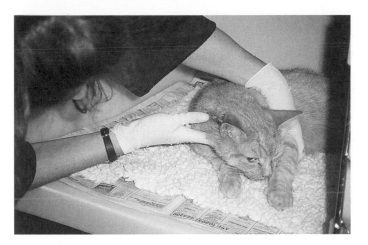

Fig. 21.6   Bedding for warmth postoperatively will support body temperature.

Temperature control

Pre- and postoperative patients need assistance to regain lost body heat and prevent the development of shock. Heat can be provided by:

- Environmental thermostat controls
- Kennels with underfloor heating
- Heated underpads (Fig. 21.6)
- Incubator for small or newborn animals

It is important never to overheat but simply to support body temperature.

Using heat lamps can be harmful if the animal is unable to move away; the animal could overheat and potentially suffer burns to the skin if the lamp is too close. Always

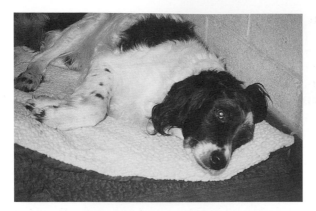

Fig. 21.7 Plenty of bedding for recumbent patients.

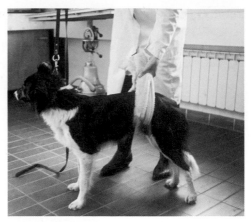

Fig. 21.8 Assist to stand using sling to support hindquarters.

keep the lamp a minimum of 1 metre from the body of the animal to avoid any overheating or burns.

Recumbent patients

- Use deep bedding to prevent pressure on any bony areas (Fig. 21.7)
- Do not allow to remain in soiled kennel
- Use incontinence pads
- Assist drinking to prevent dehydration
- Assist eating, giving small meals often
- Groom and clean away any food on the coat after feeding
- Unless contraindicated, encourage limb movements to stimulate circulation (Fig. 21.8)
- Turn the animal every 1–2 hours to prevent fluid pooling in the chest due to shallow breathing
- Rub and stroke the body to stimulate surface circulation, generating heat and fluid movement within the tissues
- Spend time playing with the animal
- Assist to urinate or check indwelling urinary catheter

Handling the hospitalised patient

Use coat care and grooming as a reason to handle. Also wipe any discharges from the nose, eye or ears and keep the area around the mouth moistened using damp cotton wool to simulate the animal's own grooming routines. This will all contribute to a feeling of well-being for the animal, accustoms them to the nursing staff and promotes recovery.

Welfare during hospitalisation

The welfare of any animal is important, but for a hospitalised patient that is absolutely dependent on its carers to meet all its needs, it is paramount. In order to address this, **nursing care plans** are now routinely used in veterinary practices. A hospitalised animal is out of its normal environment and has been admitted into an environment to which it is not used to in terms of scents, sounds and people, and so it will feel vulnerable. The behaviour of the animal may change at this time as it tries to compensate for its vulnerability. Some animals may not cope at all in this environment and will require very different care to other animals. Individualised care plans are now routinely used in veterinary practices with an aim to minimise stress for the animal and promote good welfare.

Nursing care plans are developed following an initial assessment of ten abilities of the animal which covers:

- Feeding
- Drinking
- Urination
- Defaecation
- Breathing
- Temperature
- Mobility
- Grooming
- Sleeping/resting
- Behaviour

The assessment can identify potential problems as well as actual problems, and from this information, the goals of the nursing team for the care of the animal are formulated. Once formulated, the care plan needs to be implemented by the nursing team and constantly evaluated during the time of hospitalisation for the animal. If the plan is not promoting recovery or addressing welfare concerns, then it should be adjusted accordingly.

Nursing models

In order to be effective, a nursing care plan needs to be followed systematically and included as part of a nursing model. There are a variety of nursing models in existence, and they all exist to provide the nurse with key pointers relating to patient assessment, care planning, relevant intervention, monitoring and evaluation of the patient and the nursing process.

Models follow a logical process and should be adapted to meet the patient's needs. The models to be aware of are:

- The Medical (Biomedical) Model
- The Ability Model (described earlier in formulating a care plan)

- The Roper, Logan and Tierney Model
- Orem's Model

Whichever nursing model is adopted, it is vital that all members of the nursing team are following the same processes or care is not effective. Evaluation of the nursing process is vital, particularly in cases where things do not go to plan. Animals should be seen as holistic beings, and treatment should be designed accordingly.

Isolation and barrier nursing

If the patient has a suspected contagious or zoonotic disease, it must be moved to the isolation area. Barrier nursing follows strict rules to prevent cross infection between routine patients or staff members. Barrier nursing involves:

- Wearing protective clothing – disposable apron, intact gloves and mask if necessary
- Change of footwear
- Required drugs and medical equipment for patient care
- Cleaning equipment for unit use only
- Feeding materials and cleaning of bowls in the unit
- One member of the staff to work in isolation only and not handle any other patients

Pathogenic resistance

At this point, it is pertinent to discuss pathogens that can be resistant to treatment and cause problems in the animal. Such pathogens include:

- **Methicillin-Resistant *Staphylococcus aureus* – MRSA**
  In normal circumstances, *Staphylococcus aureus* is a bacterium found on the skin surface and in the oral cavity and nasal passages of animals although a high concentration is more common in cats. In hospitalised patients, *S. aureus* can multiply and invade the body itself, causing food poisoning, skin infections and post-operative wound infections which can lead to septicaemia. *S. aureus* is a pathogen of concern as outbreaks are known to cause death. Antibiotics that are usually used to treat this bacterial infection are being seen to be ineffective in some cases due to the development of resistance within the bacteria. This resistance includes the drug methicillin, hence the term MRSA. If an outbreak is caused by MRSA, then early diagnosis and appropriate treatment are required.
- ***Clostridium difficile* – *C. difficile***
  C. difficile is a bacterium that can be found throughout the environment in soil, water, faeces and processed food products. Humans, mammals, some birds and reptiles naturally carry this bacterial strain in their intestines and suffer no effects from this. *C. difficile* can be transmitted through faeces and unknowing ingestion from

contaminated surfaces. The bacterium can produce spores that can exist in the environment for weeks/months. In the normal circumstances, if the bacterium is ingested, it is prevented from multiplying in the body by the healthy bacterial population found in the intestines. However, if an animal's healthy intestinal bacterial population is compromised due to disease or treatment with antibiotics such as penicillin and cephalosporins, then *C. difficile* takes the opportunity to multiply rapidly and cause problems by producing a toxin that attacks the lining of the intestines, leading to digestive problems and watery diarrhoea. The concern relating to *C. difficile* is that a more aggressive strain has been observed that appears to be resistant to certain treatments and has also been seen to occur in humans that have not been hospitalised or received antibiotic therapy. Research is currently being undertaken to establish whether this strain is zoonotic.

Medication

For any patient in the hospital, always check:

- Timings
- Dosage per day
- Whether tablets or injections are prescribed and whether assistance is required for successful administration
- Route

Fluid therapy

This will involve:

- Care and maintenance of intravenous catheters
- Preventing patient interference (use of Elizabethan collar)
- Checking if the fluid is running in properly
- Monitoring quantities delivered
- Changing drip fluid bags on instruction
- Monitoring hydration status
- Recording and reporting all details

Environmental enrichment

- Preferred foods
- Assisting to eat and drink; expect this to be time consuming but time well spent
- Comfort in the cage, kennel or housing
- Enough space

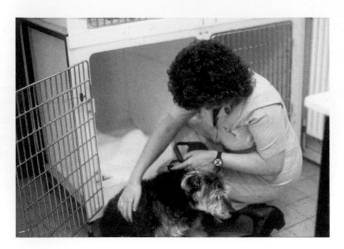

Fig. 21.9 TLC to promote recovery.

- Music helps calm both humans and animals
- Do not mix species
- Toys are helpful for long-stay patients, providing interest and, if not contraindicated, activity too
- TLC (Fig. 21.9)

Chapter 22
Monitoring Temperature, Pulse and Respiration

Summary

In this chapter, the learning outcomes are:

- To identify methods for and describe the assessment of temperature, pulse and respiration (TPR) in the animal
- To describe factors that can affect TPR assessments

The skill of observing and monitoring life signs is essential to the nursing of any species of animal. It involves the comparing of normal behaviour against that which is abnormal. Time spent with an animal, using all senses, is most important. The nurse should be capable of recognising minute changes to the animal's life signs and temperament.

Temperature, pulse and respiration or breathing can all vary in animals due to environmental temperature, recent exercise, stress situations and excitement. An increase or a decrease in the rate of these life signs can also indicate a problem with a body system or that a disease is present. These life signs should be checked hourly or, until an animal is stabilised, more frequently.

Temperature

Most species can regulate their body temperature in response to internal and external influences to within a very narrow range, due to homeostasis. Taking the body temperature of cold-blooded species like reptiles is not useful because they rely on environmental sources for their own heat. The ability of warm-blooded animals to control their own body temperature may disappear when ill or injured. Normal body temperatures for a range of mammal species are shown in Table 22.1.

Methods of losing heat from the body include:

- Sweating
- Panting

Animal Biology and Care, Third Edition. Sue Dallas and Emily Jewell.
© 2014 John Wiley & Sons, Ltd. Published 2014 by John Wiley & Sons, Ltd.
Companion Website: www.wiley.com/go/dallas/animal-biology-care

Table 22.1   Normal temperatures.

Species	Celsius	Fahrenheit
Dog	38.3–38.7	100.9–101.7
Cat	38.0–38.5	100.4–101.6
Guinea pig	38.4–40	102.2–104
Rabbit	38.5–40	101.5–104
Rat	37.5	99.9
Hamster	36–38	98–101
Mouse	37.5	99.5

- Drinking water
- Position – spread out, seeking a cold surface to lie on
- Vasodilation – surface blood vessels increase in size to lose body heat

Methods of preserving heat in the body include:

- Shivering
- Position – curled up
- Vasoconstriction – surface blood vessels reduce in size to reduce body heat loss

Temperature of the animal is assessed by:

- Touching extremities
- Body position
- Thermometer reading

Rules for assessing temperature are as follows:

- Take the temperature at the very least twice a day (it is always lower after sleep).
- Leave the thermometer in position for at least one minute; in the case of the subclinical thermometer, leave in position for at least two minutes.
- After insertion into the rectum, tilt the thermometer to contact the epithelial wall lining the tract. This ensures that the thermometer is not placed into faeces in the rectum, which would give a false reading.

Equipment required for taking an animal's temperature includes:

- Thermometer
- Lubricant such as K-Y Jelly or medicinal liquid paraffin
- Small amount of cotton wool
- Antiseptic water-based solution
- Watch with a second hand

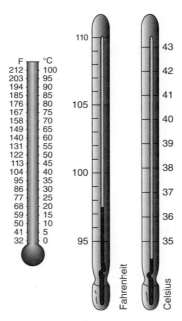

Fig. 22.1 Thermometer scales.

Process for taking an animal's temperature is as follows:

(1) Collect and prepare all required equipment.
(2) Correctly restrain patient (second person restraining the head).
(3) Prepare the thermometer to be ready to take the temperature.
(4) Apply the lubricant to the thermometer.
(5) Insert into the rectum for the correct length of time (never be tempted to reduce this time).
(6) Remove, wipe with the cotton wool and read.
(7) Wipe clean using antiseptic solution.

After the temperature has been taken:

- Store the thermometer in a jar or container containing dilute water-based antiseptic solution.
- Always wipe clean of faecal material before placing in the jar or container.
- Protect the bulb end of the thermometer by placing a layer of cotton wool at the bottom of the container.
- Never store or clean in a hot solution as this could damage the thermometer.
- Before use, wipe clean of the antiseptic solution which could irritate the rectal lining.
- Always write down the reading so that a record can be built up of any changes that occurred, at what stage of the disease and the time of day.

The types of thermometer in use include:

- Celsius or centigrade – with a scale reading of 35–43 (Fig. 22.1)
- Fahrenheit – with a scale reading of 94–108 (Fig. 22.1)
- Subclinical Celsius – with a scale reading of 25–40

The formula for converting Celsius to Fahrenheit is as follows:

F to C – subtract 32, multiply by 5, and divide by 9.
C to F – multiply by 9, divide by 5, and add 32.

Differences between:

Clinical thermometer	Laboratory thermometer	Digital thermometer
Contains mercury	Contains spirit or mercury	Digital readings
Triangular in shape	Circular in shape	Circular in shape
Scale difference	Scale difference	Fast, accurate readings
Constriction near bulb	No constriction	Use disposable cover
Needs to be shaken down before use	No shaking down before use	Check batteries charged
Short shaft	Long shaft	Hygienic

Although thermometers containing mercury have been largely superceded by digital thermometers, they may still be used in some circumstances. Care should be taken to avoid the breakage of the mercury thermometer when shaking down the mercury in preparation for reading the temperature as mercury is toxic and broken glass is hazardous.

Temperature increases may be seen:

- In infections and fevers
- After recent exercise
- In fear or excitement
- In heat stroke (*hyperthermia*)
- In hot weather

Temperature decrease may be seen:

- In shock and severe bleeding
- In exposure cases (*hypothermia*)
- In hibernation
- In anaesthesia
- Before impending death (moribund animal)
- Immediately before *parturition* (giving birth)

Pulse

The pulse is used as a means of checking the heart (*cardio*) and blood (*vascular*) function. With each heartbeat, the artery walls expand and contract in size to allow the created wave of blood to pass and maintain its speed of flow. This is called the pulse. If there is a change in the heart function or the volume of blood, then there will be a reflected change in the pulse rate (speed) or character. Normal pulse rates for a range of mammal species are shown in Table 22.2.

Table 22.2 Normal pulse recording.

Species	Pulse rate (beats per minute)
Dog	60–180*
Cat	110–180
Rabbit	150–300
Guinea pig	230–320
Hamster	300–600
Mouse	500–600

*The pulse range in dogs is due to the size variation from toy breeds (nearer the 180 end of the range) to giant breeds (nearer the 60 end of the range).

The words used to describe the pulse include:

- Intermittent
- Thready – slow, soft pulse
- Irregular
- Strong
- Weak

A normal pulse is usually described as regular, strong or firm. It is essential that time is spent feeling pulses, both normal and abnormal, to increase the operator's ability to assess the state of the animal. This will also dramatically decrease the time it takes to find the animal's pulse. The pulse can be taken where an artery runs close to the body surface. Each pulsation corresponds with the contraction of the right and left ventricles of the heart.

Sites used for taking a pulse include:

- *Femoral artery* located in the groin region on the medial aspect of the femur of the hind leg.
- *Digital artery* located on the cranial or anterior surface of the hock region of the hind leg.
- *Coccygeal artery* located on the ventral (underside) aspect of the base of the tail just above the rectum.
- *Lingual artery* located on the ventral (underside) aspect of the tongue. However, this site can only be used in unconscious or anaesthetized animals.

The most common site used to take the pulse is the femoral artery on the hind leg. Before taking the pulse, the animal must be suitably restrained so two people make the task much easier.

Taking the pulse in an animal:

(1) Ensure the animal is calmly but firmly restrained.
(2) Once the animal is settled, take the pulse by placing the fingers over the chosen artery.

(3) When properly located, using a watch with a second hand, count the pulse for one minute. Never shorten this period because the pulse can change quickly and a reading of less than one minute could be inaccurate and therefore useless.
(4) Write down the pulse count at the end of the minute.
(5) Relax the restraint of the animal and praise.

Pulse terms

- *Dysrhythmia* – indicates that the pulse and heart rate are not synchronised. The pulse is lower due to the heart pumping blood inefficiently.
- *Sinus arrhythmia* – refers to the pulse rate increase on breathing in and decrease on breathing out. This is often considered to be normal.
- *Fast pulse* – occurs when the tissues are not getting enough oxygen and the heart is compensating by speeding up to meet the body's needs. Fast pulse can be normal after exercise.

Factors that may cause a pulse increase include:

- Exercise
- Excitement or stress
- Heart/valve disease
- Shock or loss of blood
- Pain
- High temperature/fever

Factors that may cause a pulse decrease include:

- Sleep
- Unconsciousness
- Heart disease
- Other disease conditions

Respiration

Normal breathing is almost silent, although airflow may be heard in the airways. The breathing and cardiovascular systems are very closely linked, so a change in one is mirrored in the other. If the blood gas levels of oxygen or carbon dioxide become abnormal, this will be seen in the animal's colour, in its pulse rate and character and in the breathing. There should be a rhythm to the breathing, in that the time between breathing in and out should be equal. The breathing can be varied by the use of the voluntary or skeletal muscles of the chest or thorax. Normal respiration rates for a range of mammal species are shown in Table 22.3.

Certain breeds of dog and cat may, because of airway anatomy (short-nosed breeds), make considerable breathing sounds and this is normal.

The ability to voluntarily alter breathing means that the rate can only be taken once the animal has settled. Any obvious restraint will probably cause the breathing

Table 22.3 Normal respiration rates.

Species	Rate (breaths per minute)
Dog	10–30
Cat	20–30
Rabbit	35–65
Guinea pig	110–150
Hamster	75
Gerbil	90–140
Mouse	100–250

to increase in response. The reading is taken on either breathing in or breathing out and when the animal:

- Is not panting
- Has not recently exercised
- Has not been stressed by over-restraint
- Is not asleep

The respiratory rate should be taken when the animal is calm, awake and comfortable. After close observation by the operator, a decision is taken to count on breathing in or breathing out. The recording is timed using a watch with a second hand for one minute. Note is also made of the depth of breathing.

Causes of respiration increase include:

- Shock or haemorrhage
- Recent exercise
- Pain
- Excitement or fear
- Heat stroke
- Medical disease, especially of the respiratory system

Causes of respiration decrease include:

- Unconsciousness
- Sleep
- Poisons
- Low body temperature (hypothermia)

Breathing terms

- *Tachypnoea* – rapid, shallow breathing.
- *Hyperpnoea* – panting.
- *Apnoea* – no breathing taking place.
- *Cheyne–Stokes* – irregular breathing (deep breaths and then fast shallow breaths) seen shortly before death.
- *Dyspnoea* – difficulty breathing in or out and often painful.

Signs of breathing difficulties include:

- Forced breathing out
- Flaring of nostrils
- Extended head and neck
- Elbows rotated away from the chest
- Breathing through the mouth
- Exaggerated movements of the chest and abdomen
- Unusual sounds
- Unable to settle

Chapter 23
Pharmacy and the Administration of Drugs

Summary

In this chapter, the learning outcomes are:

- To define the term pharmacology
- To identify the possible routes of administration of medication in animals
- To describe the handling and dispensing of pharmacological products
- To identify and describe relevant legislation relating to veterinary medicines including:
  - Veterinary Medicines Regulations (VMR) Act 2005
  - Misuse of Drugs Regulations 1985
  - Small Animal Exemption Scheme (SAES)

Pharmacology is the branch of science concerned with the study of drugs. It covers the following aspects in relation to any drug administered to the body:

- The way in which the drug affects the body
- Absorption of the drug into the body
- Metabolism of the drug by the body
- The process of excretion of the drug from the body

The process of giving out drugs to the owner/keeper of an animal is known as *dispensing*. Drugs can either be dispensed by the veterinary practice at which the owner is registered or by taking a prescription to a dispensing chemist.

Drugs can be administered in various ways to the animal's body. The method in which the drug is administered to the body is known as the *route of administration*. The route of administration often depends on the part of the body that is the target of the drug, how quickly the effect of the drug is required and the ability of the owner to give the drug.

Animal Biology and Care, Third Edition. Sue Dallas and Emily Jewell.
© 2014 John Wiley & Sons, Ltd. Published 2014 by John Wiley & Sons, Ltd.
Companion Website: www.wiley.com/go/dallas/animal-biology-care

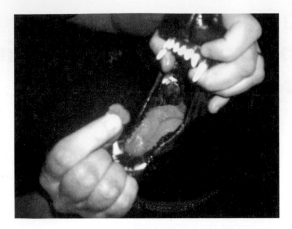

Fig. 23.1 The mouth is opened wide so that the tablet can then be placed at the back of the throat for swallowing.

Routes of administration

Oral administration (Fig. 23.1)

- This is the most frequently used route for drugs because the owner can treat at home. The products are supplied in various forms, e.g. tablet, powder, paste and liquid.
- Many tablets have an outer coating and therefore should never be broken up or crushed in case the action of the drug is reduced. Reasons for coating tablets include:
  - Protection of the drug from moisture
  - To hide an unpleasant taste
  - To assist in identification
  - To protect the drug from the hydrochloric acid in the stomach (enteric coated)
  - Protection of the stomach from the irritant effect of a drug
- Oral administration can have disadvantages:
  - If the animal is vomiting
  - Absorption can be slow and some of the drug may not be absorbed at all
  - The presence of food may reduce the drug's effect
  - The animal may refuse to swallow the drug
  - Owner is unable to give the drug to the animal

Parenteral administration

The parenteral administration route is any other administration route than the mouth. It usually refers to or is taken to mean 'by injection'. Any drug administered by this method must be sterile, and the method involves cleaning of the skin site and personal hygiene. The most frequently used injection methods are:

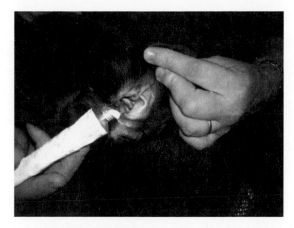

Fig. 23.2   The cream is applied to the ear flap.

 o *Subcutaneous* – into the connective tissues below the skin (below the hypodermis). This method is for non-irritant drugs, and absorption of the drug is slow.
 o *Intramuscular* – directly into a muscle body (hind leg or back). This method is used for small volumes of drug only and can be painful, but the drug is more rapidly absorbed than by the subcutaneous route.
 o *Intravenous* – into a surface vein (foreleg, hind leg or neck vein). This method places the drug directly into the bloodstream and has very rapid action.
 o Other injection routes less frequently used are:
  ■ *Epidural* – into the vertebral canal to give spinal pain control (*analgesia*)
  ■ *Intra-articular* – directly into a joint
  ■ *Intradermal* – into the skin structure

Topical administration

Drugs administered via the topical route are applied to a surface tissue of the body like the skin, eyes or ears (Fig. 23.2). They are either absorbed just into the surface of the skin or mucous membranes or the structure of the skin, depending on the material used to carry the drug. Some topical drugs may be able to move into body systems, and that is why the operator must immediately wash off any drug that contacts their skin. Types of carriers used include:

 o Water to place wettable powder against the skin
 o Petroleum jelly as ointment that melts with body heat
 o Oil and water together as a cream, which will penetrate into the skin layers
 o Detergent-based products as medicated shampoos to cover the skin surface before rinsing off

Pharmacology and dispensing

For safe drug administration, be sure that the following are checked and confirmed before medication is given:

Is it the right:

- drug?
- patient?
- dose?
- route for the drug?
- time interval?

Administering the right drug:

- Check label
- Check against the animal's medical record, if available
- If the writing is illegible on the medical record, get it clarified
- Understand the difference between trade names and generic names

Administering the right drug to the right patient:

- Check the ID on the animal
- Check the ID on the kennel
- Check any medical records

Administering the right dose:

- Read instructions
- Check with supervising member of staff

Administer the drug by the correct route:

- Know the meaning of abbreviations like:
  i.m. – intramuscular
  p.o. – by mouth (per os)
  i.v. – intravenous
  s.c. – subcutaneous
- Do not crush 'delayed action' capsules/tablets to mix with food
- Some drugs must be given i.m. for absorption as they may be irritant given s.c., so always check the instructions on the container or product leaflet

Administering the drug at the right time:

- Know the abbreviations:
  b.i.d. or b.d. – twice daily or every 12 hours
  t.i.d. or t.d. – three times daily or every 8 hours
  q.i.d. or q.d. – four times daily or every 6 hours
- Observe the drug intervals for best therapeutic levels

Any drugs given to an animal should be documented on the animal's records:

- The drug, dose, route, site of administration, date and time
- If there is no recording, assume the drug has not been given
- Record after drug is given, not before, in case of problems

Be aware of drug/food or drug/drug interactions

- Some drugs must be given with food, like aspirin
- Some drugs must be given on an empty stomach, like the antibiotic ampicillin
- Drug interactions when treating for heart disease, arthritis and epilepsy
- Record any adverse effects seen

Labels for drug containers

For legal requirements, the essential information on a container label is:

- Veterinary practice name and address
- Date of dispensing
- Owner's name and address
- The words KEEP OUT OF REACH OF CHILDREN
- The words FOR ANIMAL TREATMENT ONLY
- If applicable, the words FOR EXTERNAL USE ONLY

Additional useful information that may be included is:

- Drug strength, for example, 50 mg amoxycillin
- Trade name (licensed name for use only by the manufacturing company that developed the drug) or *generic* name (drug chemical name and manufactured by various drug companies)
- Animal's name
- Directions for use, for example, 'give twice daily'

Warnings should also be attached to certain drugs such as aspirin in full-strength form (150 mg). Labels should read 'Unsuitable for cats'. This drug can be used in humans and dogs, but in cats, its effect lasts a lot longer. If a second dose is given by the owner too soon, then the cat will be overdosed. Clearance time for aspirin is:

- Humans – 4 hours
- Dogs – 8 hours
- Cats – 30 hours

Handling and dispensing of drugs

Legal aspects

Drugs used in the treatment of animals are classified under the VMR Act of 2005 into four groups. VMR control the following aspects relating to veterinary medicines in use in the UK – manufacture, advertising, marketing, supply and administration. The VMR were updated in 2013 and came into force on 1 October 2013. Current information relating to the categorisation of medicines can be located on the Veterinary Medicine Directorate website (see further reading list):

(1) **POM-V** – these are *prescription-only medicines – veterinarian*; dispensing of these medicines can only occur once they have been prescribed by a veterinary surgeon. The veterinary surgeon must make a clinical assessment of the animal or relevant information in order to prescribe drugs in the POM-V category. POM-V drugs must be dispensed by the veterinary surgeon or a pharmacist. Examples include antimicrobials, controlled drugs (CD) and vaccinations. Some medicated feedstuffs fall into this category.

(2) **POM-VPS** – these are *prescription-only medicines – veterinary surgeons, pharmacists and suitably qualified persons (SQP)*; these medicines must be prescribed and supplied by a veterinary surgeon, pharmacist or SQP and dispensed from registered premises. A clinical assessment of the animal or relevant information is not essential to prescribe these drugs. Clients may request prescriptions to obtain the drugs elsewhere for this category of medicine. Examples of POM-VPS drugs include spot-on medications, anthelmintics and some vaccinations in farm livestock. Some medicated feedstuffs also fall into this category.

(3) **NFA-VPA** – these are *non-food animal medicines – veterinary surgeons, pharmacists and SQP*; medicines in this category are only for companion animals but not horses. These drugs must be supplied from registered premises by either a veterinary surgeon, pharmacist or SQP. A clinical assessment is not required to supply these drugs. Examples of these drugs include anthelmintics for companion animals.

(4) **AVM-GSL** – these are *authorised veterinary medicines – general sales list*; these drugs can be supplied by any retailer such as pet stores and supermarkets. Drugs in this category usually have a wide margin of safety in their usage. Examples include vitamins and minerals.

The classification group to which the medicine belongs is found on the drug container label and any outer packaging. For medicines in the POM-VPS and NFA-VPS categories, users must be advised of the safe and effective use of the medicine.

A special category of drugs, those that could be abused by humans, is known as Controlled Drugs. The legislation applicable here is the Misuse of Drugs Regulations

1985, which is divided into five schedules. These schedules are set out in decreasing order of the need to control:

- *Schedule 1* – includes drugs like cannabis and hallucinogenic drugs such as LSD, which are considered non-therapeutic and are therefore not legally held in veterinary practice for the purpose of treating animals.
- *Schedule 2* – includes the opiate analgesics (pain control) like morphine, pethidine and etorphine (anaesthetic agent). These drugs are POM, and records are kept on their ordering, supply, safe storage and, if out of date or not required, their destruction.
- *Schedule 3* – includes barbiturates (used for anaesthesia, control of epilepsy and euthanasia), some minor stimulant drugs and some analgesics (pain control). These drugs are POM and must have safe storage and purchase records.
- *Schedule 4* – includes the benzodiazepine drugs such as Valium (diazepam) (used to reduce stress). When these drugs are given to patients within the veterinary practice (e.g. in injectable form only), they are exempt from restrictions.
- *Schedule 5* – contains preparations with only traces of otherwise CD, such as cocaine, codeine (cough mixture) and morphine (kaolin and morphine for diarrhoea treatment). The levels of drug are so small that they are exempt from restrictions.

Some drugs carry special risks. Harmful products may produce an acute effect immediately after contact, whereas others may accumulate over time and constant exposure will be necessary before their effect on the operator or nurse is seen.

High-risk products include:

- Certain hormone products, like those used to postpone oestrus
- Cytotoxic drugs – those used in the treatment of cancers
- Gaseous anaesthetic agents like halothane
- Certain antibiotics
- Antifungal powders – those used to treat ringworm
- Insecticides

Small Animal Exemption Scheme

Medicines that fall into this category are those that have been licensed for use in certain pet species by the Secretary of State who has reviewed the active ingredient contained in the drug and declared that it is not required to be under veterinary control. The medicine may then be marketed under the SAES. Pets covered include aquarium fish, caged birds, homing pigeons, ferrets, rabbits, small rodents, reptiles and amphibians. Although these drugs have to be manufactured under stringent conditions and vigilantly monitored as to adverse effects and efficacy, they do not have a legal distribution category but can be similarly classed as AVM-GSL drugs.

Drugs glossary

Group	Definition
Anabolic	Promotes growth of body tissue
Analgesic	Relieves or prevents pain
Anthelmintic	Kills internal parasitic worms
Antibiotic	Disrupts or destroys bacteria
Anticoagulant	Prevents blood from clotting
Antidiuretic	Hormone which reduces urine output
Corticosteroids	Suppress inflammation
Diuretic	Increases urine production
Emetic	Causes vomiting
Sedative	Reduces awareness of surroundings
Vaccine	Stimulates the production of antibodies

Chapter 24
Isolation and Quarantine

Summary

In this chapter, the learning outcomes are:

- To identify the difference between the process of isolation and quarantine
- To describe the processes of isolation and quarantine
- To describe basic guidelines for quarantine of dogs and cats in the UK

The terms isolation and quarantine are often mistakenly interchanged, but it is important to remember that they occur at two very different times and so are separate processes.

Isolation

Isolation is required when an animal is believed to have, or has, a disease that can be passed onto others (*contagious*). There is also protective isolation for susceptible animals, e.g. unvaccinated puppies and kittens. In their case, the isolation is in the owner's home and garden, which becomes the controlled environment.

In many veterinary practices and hospitals, there is a purpose-built isolation unit where contagious animals can be housed and nursed. In other types of group housing, this type of facility may have to be created, as the need arises. Home-made isolation may involve the use of a foldaway cage or cage box in a non-animal area of the unit which can be carefully controlled.

Infectious diseases of the dog and cat needing isolation

Dog	Cat
Distemper	FIP
Hepatitis	FeLV
Leptospirosis	Feline panleucopenia
Kennel cough	Cat flu
Ringworm	Ringworm
Sarcoptic mange	

Animal Biology and Care, Third Edition. Sue Dallas and Emily Jewell.
© 2014 John Wiley & Sons, Ltd. Published 2014 by John Wiley & Sons, Ltd.
Companion Website: www.wiley.com/go/dallas/animal-biology-care

Affected animals should be housed in such a manner as to prevent other animals from coming into contact with the disease-producing organisms it will be shedding. Micro-organisms can be shed via:

- Urine
- Faeces
- Blood
- Discharges from eyes, ears, nose, mouth, prepuce, vulva or a wound
- Respiratory tract via sneezing or coughing
- Vomit

Bearing in mind the exit routes for contagious diseases, isolation must follow disease management rules:

- One member of staff specifically allocated to the isolation area
- Change into protective clothing
- Change into protective footwear or set up a footbath containing disinfectant
- Additional protection of gloves and mask
- The unit must contain all required food preparation equipment and food bowls
- Cleaning equipment to be used in the unit should be kept there
- Instruments used here are cleaned here
- Safe disposal of soiled bedding, faeces, urine, vomit, blood and saliva, which may contain infectious micro-organisms
- Required medical supplies to be available in the unit

An isolation facility must have an area for kennels, cages and a run area, for housing of various species, with a good ventilation system. Any treatments must take place within this area, which requires a sink unit, examination table and basic medical supplies. All cleaning equipment and feeding supplies for patients must be for use in isolation only. Hygiene is essential to assist the full recovery of the patient. Thorough cleaning of all surfaces, feeding equipment and bedding materials will reduce the number of micro-organisms present.

All staff members must disinfect or change footwear and overalls and wash hands in antiseptic solution before leaving to move through the other areas of the animal housing. It is essential never to put healthy animals or humans at risk by careless behaviour. There is also the possibility that the disease may transmit from animals to human carers (known as a *zoonone* or *zoonotic disease*).

Quarantine

The term quarantine refers to the detention of animals coming into the UK for a set period of time, in isolation from other animals, in order to screen for disease (Fig. 24.1). Under the Rabies Order 1974 (as amended), any animal that landed in the UK without a licence or PET passport may be directed to quarantine, exported or destroyed and its owner prosecuted. Quarantine may also be used for new animals coming into an existing animal collection.

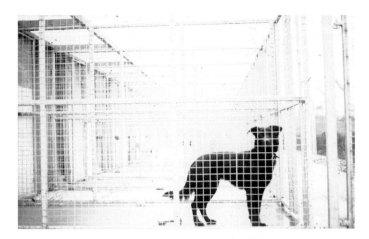

Fig. 24.1 The dog is kept isolated from others in its own housing and run area.

Quarantine time will vary depending on the species involved. For dogs and cats, the time is six calendar months to be spent in a quarantine kennel in order to screen for rabies in particular. For other species, the times and locations vary but will involve separation from the main group of animals or birds at a given location. In this manner, the resident animals are not put at risk by the newcomer.

Quarantine of dogs and cats in the UK

In March 1999, the government proposed changes to the quarantine laws, as recommended by the Kennedy Advisory Group. The Kennedy Advisory Group was appointed to look at the existing regulations and make recommendations for replacing quarantine.

The new scheme proposed to allow dogs and cats coming from EU countries, certain other European countries and rabies-free islands to enter the UK without having to undergo quarantine, provided they can meet the necessary criteria regarding vaccination and identification.

To enter the UK without quarantine from a listed or EU country, dogs and cats must have a PETS passport or certificate containing information on the animal:

- Permanently identified with an electronic microchip
- Vaccinated against rabies using an inactivated vaccine
- Have an official health certificate containing details of:
  o owner or keeper
  o identification and description of animal
  o vaccination record and booster information
  o blood tests and results
  o treatment for ticks and tapeworms

If an animal arrives in the UK and does not meet the PETS requirements (see Chapter 6), the authority responsible for carrying out the checks will decide, in consultation with the owner and a veterinary surgeon, whether to re-export the animal, to put it into quarantine (possibly for up to 6 months) until it can comply with the PETS rules or, as a last resort, to put the animal down. *See Chapter 6 for further information.*

Quarantine for 6 months on arrival in the UK should be pre-arranged before travelling begins from an unlisted country. Official transporters collect animals on arrival from ports and airports. On arrival at the quarantine premises, the animal is taken to its allocated unit. It cannot be moved to any other unit during its stay unless there is an emergency or the move is approved by the attending veterinary surgeon.

All animals are given appropriate accommodation according to size and species. There are recommended minimum internal measurements for individual units, which also state sleeping area and adjoining exercise area size.

Guidelines are in place for the general standards of hygiene and materials used on surfaces in quarantine kennels (e.g. non-slip floors). Also stated are the feeding and management routines, the need for visual stimuli and fresh air access and the condition and minimum temperature of the sleeping area.

The animal's owner is allowed reasonable access for visiting during the 6-month quarantine period. If any signs of ill health arise during the quarantine, the attending veterinary surgeon is consulted and the owner of the animal is informed immediately.

Further Reading

SECTION 1

Animal Science

Aspinall, V. & Cappello, M. (2009) *Introduction to Veterinary Anatomy and Physiology Textbook*, 2nd edition. Butterworth-Heinemann, UK.

Beckett, B. & Gallagher, R. (2001) *New Coordinated Science: Biology Students' Book: For Higher Tier*, 3rd edition. OUP, Oxford, UK.

Boden, E. (2007) *Black's Student Veterinary Dictionary*. A & C Black Publishers Ltd., London, UK.

Clegg, C.J. (2007) *Biology for the IB Diploma*. Hodder Education, UK.

Cooper, B., Mullineaux, E., & Turner, L. (2011) *BSAVA Textbook of Veterinary Nursing*, 5th edition. British Small Animal Veterinary Association (BSAVA), Gloucester, UK.

Lane, D.R., Guthrie, S., & Griffith, S. (2007) *Dictionary of Veterinary Nursing*, 3rd edition. Butterworth-Heinemann, UK.

MacKean, D.G. (2002) *Biology*, 3rd edition. Hodder Education, UK.

Masters, J. & Martin, C. (2001) *BVNA Pre-Veterinary Nursing Textbook*. Butterworth-Heinemann, UK.

Sturtz, R. & Asprea, L. (2012) *Anatomy and Physiology for Veterinary Technicians and Nurses: A Clinical Approach*. Wiley-Blackwell, UK.

Weyers, J., Reed, R., & Jones, A. (2012) *Practical Skills in Biology*, 5th edition. Pearson, UK.

Genetics

Brookes, M. (1999) *Get a Grip on Genetics*. Weidenfeld and Nicolson, London, UK.

England, G. (2012) *Dog Breeding, Whelping and Puppy Care*. Wiley Blackwell, UK.

Hollings, P. (2011) *Breeding Dogs: A Practical Guide*. The Crowood Press Ltd., UK.

Jones, S. & van Loon, B. (2011) *Introducing Genetics: A Graphic Guide*, Reprint edition. Icon Books Ltd., London, UK.

Nicholas, F.W. (2009) *Introduction to Veterinary Genetics*, 3rd edition. Wiley Blackwell, Oxford, UK.

Taylor, D. (1986) *You and Your Dog*. Dorling Kindersley, London, UK.

SECTION 2

Agar, S. (2001) *Small Animal Nutrition*. Butterworth Heinnemann, London, UK.

Alderton, D. (1997) *The Reptile Survival Manual*. Ringpress Books, Gloucestershire, UK.

Animal Biology and Care, Third Edition. Sue Dallas and Emily Jewell.
© 2014 John Wiley & Sons, Ltd. Published 2014 by John Wiley & Sons, Ltd.
Companion Website: www.wiley.com/go/dallas/animal-biology-care

Alderton, D. (2011a) *The Ultimate Encyclopedia of Caged & Aviary Birds: A Practical Family Reference Guide to Keeping Pet Birds*. Southwater, London, UK.

Alderton, D. (2011b) *Encyclopedia of Aquarium & Pond Fish*. Dorling Kindersley, London, UK.

Alderton, D. (2012) *The Ultimate Encyclopedia of Small Pets & Pet Care*. Southwater, London, UK.

Alderton, D., Edwards, A., & Stockman, M. (2011) *The Complete Book of Pets & Petcare*. Southwater, London, UK.

Anderson, R.S. & Edney, A.T.B. (1990) *Practical Animal Handling*. Pergamon Press, Oxford, UK.

Bradshaw, J., Brown, S.L., & Casey, R. (2012) *The Behaviour of the Domestic Cat*, 2nd edition. CABI Publishing, Oxfordshire, UK.

Broom, D.M (1991) Animal Welfare: Concepts and measurements, *Journal of Animal Science* 69, 4168.

Brown, M. & Richardson, V. (2000) *Rabbitlopaedia: A Complete Guide to Rabbit Care*. Ringpress Books, Dorking, UK.

Burger, I. (1993) *The Waltham Book of Companion Animal Nutrition*. Pergamon Press, Oxford, UK.

Cannon, M. & Forster-van Hijfte, M. (2006) *Feline Medicine: A Practical Guide for Veterinary Nurses and Technicians*. Butterworth-Heinemann, London, UK.

Colville, J. & Berryhill, D. (2007) *Handbook of Zoonoses: Identification and Prevention*. Mosby, St. Louis, MO.

Cooper, B., Mullineaux, E., & Turner, L. (2011) *BSAVA Textbook of Veterinary Nursing*, 5th edition. British Small Animal Veterinary Association, Gloucester, UK.

Dallas, S. & Simpson, G. (1999) *Manual of Veterinary Care*. BSAVA, Gloucester, UK.

Dallas, S., North, D., & Angus, J. (2006) *Grooming Manual for the Dog and Cat*. Wiley-Blackwell, Oxford, UK.

DEFRA (2013) Taking your pet abroad [Online]. Available at: https://www.gov.uk/take-pet-abroad. Accessed on 28 September 2013.

Ducommum, D. (2011) *Rats: Practical, Accurate Advice from the Expert (Complete Care Made Easy)*. Bow Tie Press, Irvine, CA.

Edney, A. (2006) *RSPCA Complete Cat Care Manual*. Dorling Kindersley, London, UK.

Elward, M. & Ruelokke, M. (2003) *Guinea Piglopaedia: A Complete Guide to Guinea Pigs*. Interpet Publishing, London, UK.

England, G. & von Heimendahl, A. (2010) *BSAVA Manual of Reproduction and Neonatology*, 2nd edition. British Small Animal Veterinary Association, Gloucester, UK.

Evans, J.M. & White, K. (1994a) *Book of the Bitch*. Henston, Guildford, UK.

Evans, J.M. & White, K. (1994b) *The Catlopaedia*. Henston, Guildford, UK.

Evans, J.M. & White, K. (1994c) *The Doglopaedia*. Henston, Guildford, UK.

Fogle, B. (2006) *RSPCA Complete Dog Care Manual*. Dorling Kindersley, London, UK.

Fogle, B. (2011) *Complete Cat Care: What Every Cat Owner Needs to Know*. Mitchell Beazley, London, UK.

Gay, J. (2005) *The Perfect Aquarium: The Complete Guide to Setting up and Maintaining an Aquarium*. Hamlyn, London, UK.

Girling, S.J. (2013) *Nursing of Exotic Pets*, 2nd edition. Wiley-Blackwell, West Sussex, UK.

Gunn, A. & Pitt, S.J. (2012) *Parasitology: An Integrated Approach*. Wiley Blackwell, Chichester, UK.

Gurney, P. (2011) *Guinea Pig (Collins Family Pet Guide)*, Relaunch edition. HarperCollins.

Harkness, J.E. & Wagner, J.E. (1985) *The Biology and Medicine of Rabbits and Rodents*. Lea & Febiger, Philadelphia, PA.

Harvey, A. & Tasker, S. (2013) *BSAVA Manual of Feline Practice: A Foundation Manual*. British Small Animal Veterinary Association, Gloucester, UK.

Horwitz, D. & Mills, D.S. (2010) *BSAVA Manual of Canine and Feline Behavioural Medicine*. BSAVA, Gloucester, UK.

Hotston-Moore, P. & Hughes, A. (2007) *Manual of Practical Animal Care*. British Small Animal Veterinary Association, Gloucester, UK.

International Cat Care (2013a) *Feline Immunodeficiency Virus* [Online]. Available at: http://www.icatcare.org/advice-centre/cat-health/feline-immunodeficiency-virus-fiv. Accessed on 14 September 2013.

International Cat Care (2013b) *Feline Infectious Anaemia* [Online]. Available at: http://www.icatcare.org/advice-centre/cat-health/feline-haemoplama-infectiouns-feline-infectious-anaemia-0. Accessed on 14 September 2013.

International Cat Care (2013c) *Feline Infectious Peritonitis* [Online]. Available at: http://www.icatcare.org/advice-centre/cat-health/feline-infectious-peritonitis-fip. Accessed on 14 September 2013.

International Cat Care (2013d) *Feline Leukaemia Virus* [Online]. Available at: http://www.icatcare.org/advice-centre/cat-health/feline-leukaemia-virus-felv. Accessed on 14 September 2013.

Keeble, E. & Meredith, A. (2009) *BSAVA Manual of Rodents and Ferrets*. BSAVA, Gloucester, UK.

Laber-Laird, K., Flecknell, P., & Swindle, M. (1996) *Handbook of Rodent and Rabbit Medicine*. Butterworth-Heinemann, London, UK.

Lane, D.R., Guthrie, S., & Griffith, S. (2007) *Dictionary of Veterinary Nursing*, 3rd edition. Butterworth-Heinemann, London, UK.

Logsdail, C., Logsdail, P., & Hovers, K. (2003) *Hamsterlopaedia*. Ringpress Books Ltd., Dorking, UK.

Meredith, A. & Johnson Delaney, C. (2010) *BSAVA Manual of Exotic Pets*, 5th edition. British Small Animal Veterinary Association, Gloucester, UK.

Morris, D. (1986) *Animal Watching*. Jonathan Cape, London, UK.

PFMA (2012) *Pet Population* [Online]. Available at: http://www.pfma.org.uk/pet-population/. Accessed on 6 May 2013.

Smith, J. (2012) *Rats – Pet Friendly*. Magnet & Steel Publishing Ltd., London, UK.

Sandford, G. (2004) *Mini Encyclopaedia of the Tropical Aquarium*, Interpet Publishing, Dorking, UK.

Taylor, D. (2002) *Collins Small Pet Handbook: Looking After Rabbits, Hamsters, Guinea-Pigs, Gerbils, Mice and Rats*, Collins.

Tynes, V. (2010) *Behavior of Exotic Pets*. Wiley-Blackwell, Chichester, UK.

Vanderlip, S. (2003) *The Guinea-Pig Handbook*. Barron's Educational Series, New York.

Varga, M., Lumbis, R., & Gott, L. (2012) *BSAVA Manual of Exotic Pet and Wildlife Nursing*. British Small Animal Veterinary Association, Gloucester, UK.

Warren, D. (2009) *Small Animal Care and Management*, 3rd edition. Delmar, CA.

SECTION 3

Aldridge, P. & O'Dwyer, L. (2013) *Practical Emergency and Critical Care Veterinary Nursing*, Wiley-Blackwell, Chichester, UK.

Aspinall, V. (2008) *Clinical Procedures in Veterinary Nursing*, 2nd edition. Butterworth-Heinemann, London, UK.

Aspinall, V. (2012) *The Complete Textbook of Veterinary Nursing*, 2nd edition. Butterworth-Heinemann, London, UK.

Boldrick, L. (2010) *Essential First Aid for Dog Owners*. All Publishing Company, Orange, CA.

BSAVA (2013) *Medicines Classification* [Online]. Available at: http://www.bsava.com/Advice/BSAVAGuidetotheUseofVeterinaryMedicines/Medicinesclassification/tabid/352/Default.aspx. Accessed on 4 October 2013.

Colville, J. & Oien, S. (2013) *Clinical Veterinary Language*. Mosby, St. Louis, MO.

Cooper, B., Mullineaux, E., & Turner, L. (2011) *BSAVA Textbook of Veterinary Nursing*, 5th edition. BSAVA British Small Animal Veterinary Association, Gloucester, UK.

Edney, A.T.B. & Hughes, I.B. (1986) *Pet Care*. Blackwell Science, Oxford, UK.

Fogle, B. (1995) *First Aid for Dogs*. Pelham, London, UK.

McBride, D.F. (1996) *Learning Veterinary Terminology*. Mosby, St. Louis, MO.

Orpet, H. & Welsh, P. (2010) *Handbook of Veterinary Nursing*, 2nd edition. Wiley-Blackwell, UK.

Taylor, D. (1986) *You and Your Cat*. Dorling Kindersley, London, UK.

VMD (2013) *Information for veterinary professionals* [Online]. Available at: http://www.vmd.defra.gov.uk/vet.aspx. Accessed on 4 October 2013.

Appendix
Anatomy and Physiology Terminology

The majority of terms referring to the body systems and medical conditions are derived from Greek or Latin. Most of these terms are a combination of two or more word parts. When they combine to become a word, they usually indicate some or all of the following:

- Body tissues involved
- What has gone wrong
- Quantity (a lot or very little)
- Levels of infection or inflammation
- Colour or substance
- Fluid involved

You may find it helpful to practise defining the components of the words separately and then combine them to find out the meaning of the complete word. In many ways, it is no different from learning a new language, and by memorizing the common beginnings and endings, the rest can be worked out. It is always helpful to have a veterinary dictionary for the less frequently used terms and words.

Medical terminology

Certain syllables are commonly used as the beginning or ending of medical terms, in many cases being added to a word stem which refers to a particular organ or part of the body:

- *Prefix* – beginning of a word stem
- *Suffix* – ending of a word stem

Animal Biology and Care, Third Edition. Sue Dallas and Emily Jewell.
© 2014 John Wiley & Sons, Ltd. Published 2014 by John Wiley & Sons, Ltd.
Companion Website: www.wiley.com/go/dallas/animal-biology-care

Prefixes in anatomy/physiology

A or **An** – lack of, e.g. anaemia (lack of blood cells)
Dys – difficult or defective, e.g. dysphagia (difficulty swallowing)
Endo – within, e.g. endoscope (equipment used to look at working organs)
Ex – out, e.g. excision (to remove)
Haema or **Haemo** – refers to blood, e.g. haemorrhage (loss of blood)
Hyper – excess of, e.g. hyperthermia (high body temperature)
Hypo – lack of, e.g. hypothermia (low body temperature)
Poly – many or much, e.g. polydipsia (drinking a lot)
Pyo – pus, e.g. pyometra (pus-filled uterus)
Sub – beneath or under, e.g. sublingual (under the tongue)

Suffixes in anatomy/physiology

itis – inflammation, e.g. arthritis (inflammation of a joint)
logy – science or study of, e.g. dermatology (study of the skin)
penia – deficiency, e.g. leucopenia (deficiency of white blood cells)
phagia – eating, e.g. coprophagia (eating faeces)
rrhoea – increased discharge, e.g. diarrhoea (increased discharge of faeces)

Word use

The following common words may help to illustrate the prefix/suffix idea:

* *Nephritis* – **neph** refers to the specialized cell of the kidney, known as the nephron; **itis** refers to the inflammation of a tissue. The meaning of this word is kidney cell inflammation and pain.
* *Arthritis* – **arth** refers to a joint; **itis** means inflammation. The meaning of this word is joint inflammation and pain.
* *Hepatitis* – **hepat** refers to the specialized cell of the liver known as the hepatocyte; **itis** means inflammation. This word means inflammation and pain of the liver cells.
* *Haematoma* – **haem** refers to blood; **toma** refers to a lump or swelling. The meaning of this word is blood-filled lump or swelling.

These words are descriptions, not diagnoses, and simply refer to a tissue type or organ and what is happening to it.

Anatomical directions

Anatomical directions are used to describe areas of the animal body (Fig. A.1). They are part of the language of medicine used between colleagues for communication. Many of these words originated from Greek or Latin.

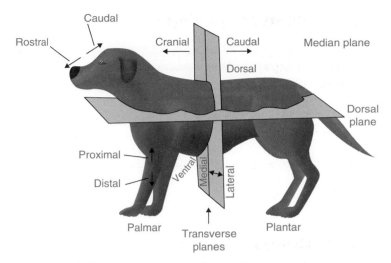

Fig. A.1 Anatomical directions. Source: Adapted from McBride, D.F. (1996) *Learning Veterinary Terminology.* Reproduced with permission of Elsevier.

The first four words are another way of saying above, below, front and back and are in common use when case recording in the medical world:

- *Dorsal* – towards the top or back surface of the body
- *Ventral* – towards the underside, lower surface or nearer the ground
- *Cranial or anterior* – situated at the front of the body or towards the head end
- *Caudal or posterior* – situated towards the back end of the body or towards the tail

Words to indicate side, middle or near the nose are:

- *Lateral* – to the side (left or right) or away from the middle of the body
- *Medial* – the midline of a body structure or the body
- *Rostral* – on the head but towards the nose

Words indicating near or far from a named body structure (especially limbs) are:

- *Proximal* – near to the body trunk or closer to a named structure
- *Distal* – away from the body trunk or further from a named structure

Words which describe where on a limb, surface, especially lower limb, surfaces are:

- *Palmar or volar* – indicating the caudal or back surface of the forelimb, below the carpus or wrist area

- *Plantar* – indicating the caudal or back surface of the hindlimb, below the tarsus or hock area

Words indicating inside or outside are:

- *Internal* – inside the body
- *External* – outside or surface

Index

Note: Page numbers in *italics* refer to Figures; those in **bold** to Tables.

Animal Biology and Care, Third Edition. Sue Dallas and Emily Jewell.
© 2014 John Wiley & Sons, Ltd. Published 2014 by John Wiley & Sons, Ltd.
Companion Website: www.wiley.com/go/dallas/animal-biology-care